Lecture Notes of the Institute for Computer Sciences, Social Informatics and Telecommunications Engineering

485

The LNICST series publishes ICST's conferences, symposia and workshops.
LNICST reports state-of-the-art results in areas related to the scope of the Institute.
The type of material published includes

- Proceedings (published in time for the respective event)
- Other edited monographs (such as project reports or invited volumes)

LNICST topics span the following areas:

- General Computer Science
- E-Economy
- E-Medicine
- Knowledge Management
- Multimedia
- Operations, Management and Policy
- Social Informatics
- Systems

José Manuel Machado · Hugo Peixoto
Editors

AI-assisted Solutions for COVID-19 and Biomedical Applications in Smart Cities

Third EAI International Conference, AISCOVID-19 2022
Braga, Portugal, November 16–18, 2022
Proceedings

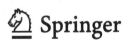

Springer

Editors
José Manuel Machado
University of Minho
Braga, Portugal

Hugo Peixoto
University of Minho
Braga, Portugal

ISSN 1867-8211 ISSN 1867-822X (electronic)
Lecture Notes of the Institute for Computer Sciences, Social Informatics
and Telecommunications Engineering
ISBN 978-3-031-38203-1 ISBN 978-3-031-38204-8 (eBook)
https://doi.org/10.1007/978-3-031-38204-8

This Springer imprint is published by the registered company Springer Nature Switzerland AG
The registered company address is: Gewerbestrasse 11, 6330 Cham, Switzerland

Preface

We are delighted to introduce the proceedings of the third edition of the EAI AISCOVID-19, International Conference on AI-assisted Solutions for COVID-19 and Biomedical Applications in Smart-Cities. This conference brought together researchers, developers, and practitioners around the world who are leveraging and developing AI-assisted technology for a smarter and more robust healthcare domain. The theme of AISCOVID-19 2022 was "Healthcare effective and efficient Solutions for COVID-19 that can be achieved using Artificial Intelligence and Computer-Assisted paradigms".

Whether you are a healthcare professional, a data scientist, or simply interested in the role of technology in healthcare, this book offers a comprehensive and up-to-date look at the intersection of COVID-19, big data, machine learning, deep learning, and healthcare.

The technical program of AISCOVID-19 2022 consisted of 8 full papers at the main conference tracks. The conference tracks were: The conference was held fully online but the discussion and technical level of the presentations was impressive, making a huge impact on the overall participants.

Coordination with the steering chairs, Imrich Chlamtac, Juan Pavón from Universidad Complutense Madrid, and Vicente Julian from Universitat Politècnica de València was essential for the success of the conference. We sincerely appreciate their constant support and guidance. It was also a great pleasure to work with such an excellent organizing committee team for their hard work in organizing and supporting the conference. In particular, the Technical Program Committee, led by our TPC Chairs, José Luis Calvo Rolle, Gianni Vercelli and the TPC co-Chairs Deden Jacob, and Ichiro Satoh, and all the reviewers completed the peer-review process of technical papers and made a high-quality technical program. We are also grateful to Conference Manager Kristína Havlíčková for her support and to all the authors who submitted their papers to the AISCOVID19 2022 conference.

We strongly believe that AISCOVID-19 2022 provided a good forum for all researchers, developers and practitioners to discuss all science and technology aspects that are relevant to the main topics of this volume. We also expect that the future AISCOVID conferences will be as successful and stimulating, as indicated by the contributions presented in this volume.

November 2022

José Manuel Machado
Hugo Peixoto

Organization

Steering Committee

Imrich Chlamtac	University of Trento, Italy
Juan Pavón	Universidad Complutense Madrid, Spain
Vicente Julian	Universitat Politècnica de València, Spain

Organizing Committee

General Chair

José Machado — University of Minho, Portugal

General Co-Chair

Hugo Peixoto — University of Minho, Portugal

TPC Chairs

José Luis Calvo Rolle	University of la Coruña, Spain
Gianni Vercelli	Università di Genova, Italy

TPC Co-Chairs

Deden Jacob	Telkom University, Indonesia
Ichiro Satoh	National Institute of Informatics, Japan

Sponsorship and Exhibit Chair

Dalila Durães — University of Minho, Portugal

Local Chairs

Daniela Oliveira	University of Minho, Portugal
Ailton Moreira	University of Minho, Portugal

Workshops Chairs

António Abelha   University of Minho, Portugal
Hector Alaiz Moreton   University of Leon, Spain
Paulo Novais   University of Minho, Portugal

Publicity and Social Media Chairs

Diana Ferreira   University of Minho, Portugal
Cristiana Neto   University of Minho, Portugal

Publications Chairs

Nicolas Lori   University of Minho, Portugal
Júlio Duarte   University of Minho, Portugal

Web Chairs

Regina Sousa   University of Minho, Portugal
Rui Miranda   University of Minho, Portugal

Posters and PhD Track Chair

Fernando Moreira   Universidade Portucalense, Portugal

Panels Chairs

Hélia Guerra   University of the Azores, Portugal
Luís Mendes Gomes   University of the Azores, Portugal

Demos Chair

Hélia Guerra   University of the Azores, Portugal

Tutorials Chairs

Hélia Guerra   University of the Azores, Portugal
Gianni Vercelli   University of Genoa, Italy

Contents

COVID-19 Global Impact

Not Necessarily Relaxed: How Work Interruptions Affect Users' Perception of Stress in Remote Work Situations

Lukas Metzger[✉], Aaron Kutzner, and Karsten Huffstadt

University of Applied Sciences Würzburg-Schweinfurt, Faculty of Computer Science and Business Information Systems, Sanderheinrichsleitenweg 20, 97074 Würzburg, Germany

{lukas.metzger,aaron.kutzner}@student.fhws.de, lu.metz@icloud.com, karsten.huffstadt@fhws.de

Abstract. Remote work was ubiquitous during the COVID-19 pandemic to minimize the spread of the virus. However, working away from the actual workplace also presented new challenges. In a study conducted in 2020, a research team from Switzerland examined the effects of acute work stress in a group office setting. Part of the study included examining the effects of work interruptions. We took this as an opportunity to conduct an exploratory study of the subjective perception of work interruptions during remote work regarding stress. Using eye-tracking technology, we investigated the visual attention of subjects within a laboratory experiment while they were repeatedly interrupted while performing a work task. We then processed the experiences in qualitative interviews to reconstruct the social reality of the effects of remote work interruptions. According to our results, we assume that the more personal standards cannot be met in case of interruptions, the stronger the subjective stress experience. This should be further explored in quantitative studies. We were able to draw up further findings in the form of recommendations to managers. For example, unnecessary interruptions should be minimized, or better yet, eliminated. Alternatively, necessary work interruptions should be directed to employees who appear to have more capacity to respect and protect the concentration of busy employees. We hope that further research will follow up on this topic in the future. In this way, robust approaches that promote the mental health of employees in the home office can be formulated to avoid unnecessary stressors, and contribute to effectiveness, efficiency, and well-being.

Keywords: Eye-Tracking · Work Stress · Remote Work

1 Introduction

1.1 Current Situation

Remote working became an integral part of everyday working life in Germany in 2020, 2021 and 2022. After the German Infectious Diseases Protection Act came

ICST Institute for Computer Sciences, Social Informatics and Telecommunications Engineering 2023
Published by Springer Nature Switzerland AG 2023. All Rights Reserved
J. M. Machado and H. Peixoto (Eds.): AISCOVID 2022, LNICST 485, pp. 3–15, 2023.
https://doi.org/10.1007/978-3-031-38204-8_1

into force in March 2020, which primarily served to contain the consequences of the COVID-19 pandemic, 27% of all employees nationwide were already working mostly from home according to a representative survey of employees in April 2020 [3]. Despite sometimes considerable adverse circumstances such as technical incidents and family care problems, 74% of all respondents were either satisfied or even very satisfied with the new, flexible working conditions [4]. Due to increasing digitization and new work approaches, remote work is a phenomenon that deserves special attention. In particular, the effects on employees whose daily work routine have changed in recent years or will change in the future should be researched. A field of research, generated and driven by the digital transformation, gives rise to a closer look in many respects.

1.2   Related Work

In a previous stress study which was conducted in Switzerland, a research team investigated the effects of acute work stress in open-plan offices [6]. They evaluated the psychobiological stress reactions, which were measured by changes in salivary cortisol and salivary alpha-amylase as well as heart rate, and the cognitive assessment of the psychosocial stress test. For this research, the Trier Social Stress Test (TSST) according to Kirschbaum et al. from 1993 [7] was used. They were able to show that the group of participants who, in addition to psychosocial stress, were additionally interrupted in their tasks, showed a higher increase in cortisol levels than the group without induced work interruptions. Work interruptions are among the most important stressors in the workplace [13]. Surprisingly, participants in the group with work interruptions rated themselves calmer and in better mood, in contradiction to increased psychobiological stress responses. Therefore, there was no correlation between increased physiological stress and psychological stress perception [6].

That this aspect need not be surprising at all has already been established in an earlier study from 2012 that examined over 358 TSST and TSST-related studies published in pubMed between 1993 and August 2011 [1]. These were systematically reviewed for the relationship between participants' physiological responsiveness to acute stress and subjective reports of affective experience. The researchers reasoned that TSST has been repeatedly shown to reliably stimulate the hypothalamic-pituitary-adrenocortical (HPA) axis and trigger cardiovascular responses, but too little attention has been paid to subjective feelings of stress at this time. Moreover, cognitive, and emotional processes are considered to be the main pathways in triggering the arousal of negative physiological states and thus causing long-term pathological health conditions.

Specifically, Campbell and Ehlert's study [1] examined stress-induced biological and emotional stress responses for a correlation or predictive relationship. Three inclusion criteria were considered: (1) exposure to the standard TSST or slightly modified versions, (2) at least one assessment of subjective emotional stress experience before, during, or after the TSST, (3) reported correlations between acute physiological as well as emotional stress measures. Attention to these aspects led to a cluster of 49 studies, which were then examined in more detail. It was concluded that significant correlations between cortisol responses and perceived emotional stress variables were found in only about 25% of the studies [1].

Furthermore, the "Transactional Stress Model" of Lazarus and Folkman from 1984 provides information about the development of subjective stress perception. According to this model, stress is caused by a stimulus that hits a person from the environment. This is only classified as stress if the individual considers it to be dangerous and if there is also a lack of resources (e.g., lack of time). However, with the help of a suitable coping strategy, an initially stressful situation can also be re-evaluated under the presence of certain aspects [9]. In addition, Ursin and Eriksen emphasize in their cognitive activation theory from 2004 that the subjective experience of stress results from the evaluation of a perceived stimulus as harmful or threatening [12].

1.3 Research Objective

In times of increasing remote work, this study aims to investigate the extent to which digital work interruptions are perceived in terms of subjective stress. Due to the patchy state of studies on this topic, the question arises as to how this form of work stressors affects people and why an interruption is classified as stress.

The research thus aims to reconstruct the perception of work interruptions regarding the perception of stress during remote work and to derive a hypothesis from this, which should be examined in more detail in further studies. This should help to further advance stress research with reference to digital work.

2 Methodology

In 2020, Kerr et. al. studied the effects of acute work stress in a group office environment and evaluated the psychobiological stress responses of subjects during presence work. In an experiment, a work situation was created that was as real as possible in an open-plan office. Stress reactivity was then measured via interviews and saliva tests [6]. Furthermore, since the literature so far has mostly provided quantitative research results regarding work interruptions and remote work, the research question in this paper was approached exploratively and qualitatively.

The methodology consisted of two parts: First, we induced a classic remote work situation using a laboratory experiment. We combined this with an eye-tracking study to record the visual attention of the subjects and to support our qualitative research with the results. We then used qualitative interviews to reconstruct the social reality of digital working. Specifically with the experiment, we ensured that the following interviews could address the experiences and perceptions of what was experienced. We decided against research based purely on qualitative interviews. So we avoid the possibility that people away from their remote workplace and outside their working hours would assess the impact of work interruptions and accompanying stressors differently. The laboratory experiment including eye-tracking was first conducted with all subjects. Immediately after the experiment, the interviews were conducted to be able to directly address the still fresh experiences.

2.1 Laboratory Experiment and Eye-Tracking

First, six subjects were invited to participate in the experiment. In order not to falsify the results of the interviews, no one was told in advance what the actual goal of the research experiment was and that the interview would be conducted afterwards. The research was disguised in advance as an eye-tracking study, the content was the analysis of an English text.

Experiment and Work Situation. During the laboratory experiment all test persons received the same task by mail: They should prepare a pitch for a presentation on Information Security Awareness (ISA). This should take place digitally via Zoom and be presented to a local institute. The background is that employees of the institute are to be trained on ISA. The presentation is to be supported with the help of a paper on the topic of ISA training via virtual reality [5]. This served as essential source material so that subjects did not have to search the Internet for information themselves. Specifically, the subjects were asked to summarize and present the main statements and the hard facts of the paper on three to four slides. To do this, they did not have to read the entire paper, but rather compile the key findings in the results section. All subjects had 30 min. Afterwards, the results were to be presented via Zoom. The task was not intended to be too difficult, but challenging, so that the subjects were busy for this time. The experiment took place on the premises of the University of Applied Sciences Würzburg-Schweinfurt in the institute building of the Faculty of Computer Science and Business Information Systems. Here, an equal laboratory environment could be provided for all test persons. As usual for a remote working situation, the main working tools were a notebook and a smartphone. Additionally, a DIN-A4 letter pad and a ballpoint pen for handwritten notes were provided (see. Fig. 1). During the experiment, the participants were exposed to the usual influences of a remote work situation. These were interruptions by short phone calls and small work tasks to be completed in between. During the interruptions, subjects were told that a creative presentation was to be made by the presenter in the upcoming Zoom meeting. For this, the participants were to compose and send mails with personal information for the alleged moderator.

Eye-Tracking. During the performance of the work task, all subjects wore eye-tracking glasses. The model used was the Glasses 2 from the manufacturer Tobii. The eye-tracking technology was used to clarify further questions in addition to the findings from the interviews. While in the interviews purely the subjective sensations of the participants could be discussed, eye-tracking allowed to

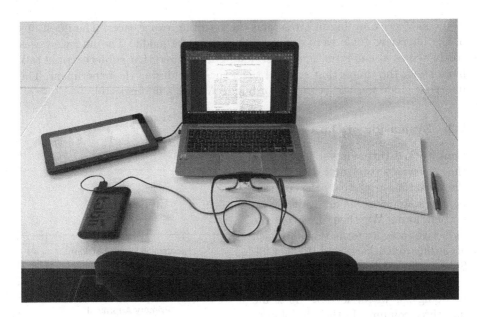

Fig. 1. Test Setup: Notebook, Tobii Glasses 2 and Writing Materials

precisely document the visual attention during the experiment. Based on this, a better understanding of the individuals' approach can be formed. Attention before, during, and after the interruptions could be recorded, thus underpinning and enriching findings from the interviews. Two aspects could be illuminated with the help of eye-tracking:

- Impairment of visual attention during interruptions
- Influencing the continuation of the actual main task

2.2 Qualitative Interviews

After 30 min working on their main task, the participants received an e-mail with an invitation to a Zoom meeting in which they were to dial in. Once they were in the meeting, the eye-tracking recording was stopped and backed up. Subjects then were allowed to remove their glasses. To avoid confusion, the participants were now informed that there would be no pitch, but that an interview would be conducted about their experiences within the experiment as well as about their everyday digital professional life. After the participants agreed, the interview was recorded, and the processing of the interview guide was carried out. Through the interviews the subjective feelings of the disruptions related to the actual task objective were discussed. The interview guide was constructed using the transactional stress model (see Fig. 2) of Lazarus and Folkman from 1984 [9]. This provided the basis for elaborating the perception of the situation in terms of the subjective feeling of stress and the resulting experiences. The questions of the interview guide were derived from the stress model. The interview was conducted as a semi-structured interview. This ensured that subjects could talk more about the things that stressed them the most during the experiment. The interview guide was structured according to Misoch's findings [10].

2.3   Evaluation of Data

Qualitative Interviews. To analyze the interviews, we first transcribed the recordings so that the participants' statements were available in textual form. We then drew on the inductive category formation approach according to Kuckartz and Rädiker [8]. Specifically, we used the concept of category formation via focused summary. In doing so, we divided a .docx file into three columns. In the left column, we inserted the original transcript. In the middle column, we summarized the statements of the participants to form superordinate categories and associated subcategories in the right column. By means of assignment, we were then able to assign further text passages either to categories or subcategories or to merge them.

Eye-Tracking. The recordings, which were made during the experiment using eye-tracking, were evaluated by visual observation. Usually, heatmaps or gaze plots are suitable for the representation of visual attention. However, these forms of visualization were not suitable for our use case because the observation involved very dynamic work, rather than simply viewing a static image or website. In Sect. 2.1. we already mentioned the main research content for which we used eye-tracking. During the visual observation of the recordings, we observed the sections in which the subjects were interrupted in their work, as well as the time

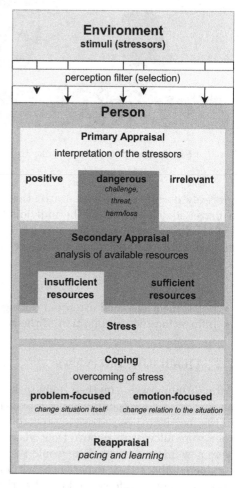

Fig. 2. Own Presentation of Lazarus' and Folkmans Stress Model [9]

before and after the interruptions. We summarized in a table which participant was working on what and how the interruptions affected the visual attention and the actual processing of the main task.

3 Results and Discussion

In the following, we first state the hypothesis H and justify it based on our findings from the eye-tracking recordings and the interviews. Subsequently, we address further effects of interruptions on individuals and present possible recommendations R1 and R2 for managers and decision makers.

3.1 Hypothesis and Justifications

As a result of our work, after analyzing the data, we were able to formulate and justify the following hypothesis H.

H: The more personal standards cannot be met in the event of an interruption, the stronger the subjective stress experience is.

Through the interviews we learned that the independent and autonomous processing of a task is always determined by the individuals' own standards or goals - especially in remote work situations.

These standards are:

- Quality
- Strategy/structure or planning/approach
- Self-actualization or perfectionism
- Focus
- Safety mechanisms

Depending on the severity of the interruption, the adherence to these personal standards is disturbed. The subjective stress experience then does not occur directly through the interruption, but through the consequences regarding the non-compliance with one's own standards. For example, the quality can be curbed by the resulting time pressure. Especially if a work result is expected at a certain point in time with a certain quality (e.g., a presentation to a committee), the lack of time becomes a threat to this goal. Consequently, due to the interruption and possibly additional tasks, the own quality standard of the main task must be lowered. The processing is then no longer carried out with the same accuracy.

In addition, the disruption can mean that the own strategy or approach to a task can no longer be adhered to. Remote work is characterized by employees organizing themselves. Therefore, it is necessary to bring structure into the daily work routine. This was also reported by the study participants. Often, there are only framework conditions that must be adhered to. These include, for example, the specific work tasks and goals to be achieved, as well as deadlines for completion. The time at which the work is to be completed, as well as tools or, if necessary, people who can give tips on how to complete the work, are often freely selectable. Once the workday has been planned and deadlines have been set, there are time frames for the independent processing of the work content. However, if these cannot be used, or at least not optimally, due to interruptions and additional tasks, rescheduling is necessary. This is in contradiction to the original planning. The feeling that the specially planned structure for the workday has been partially or even completely wasted is classified as a subjective feeling of stress. It is similar with the perfectionism of a person with its work. In addition to the expected work result, employees also want to realize themselves in their work and therefore also have their own demand for a perfect result of their work. If this wish cannot be fulfilled due to interruptions and the resulting lack of time, psychological stress also results.

In addition, there is the personal focus. People want to work effectively and efficiently. However, this is only possible with the right focus - especially in the home office. It is therefore important to concentrate on different aspects of a task for a certain period and to focus one's attention only on these aspects. We put this to the test in our experiment. The course of the subjects' focus became comprehensible by recording their visual attention via eye-tracking. For example, we were able to observe the extent to which interruptions interfered with the processing of the task. It became clear that the more interruptions the participants had, the more difficult it was for them to find their way back into the task. This could be seen in the fact that text sections had to be read several times after an interruption. In some cases, the subjects also changed subtasks and decided to work on a different subtask after they had been interrupted. If they were in the process of summarizing a text section in handwritten bullet points shortly before the interruption, they did not continue with it after the interruption and opened, for example, a program for creating the slides. This again contradicts the personal structuring of a task, so that subtasks are processed one after the other. This was described as an enormous burden, since a great deal of concentration was required to refind the task. A lot of mental resources had to be expended to continue with the main task in a focused manner after the interruptions.

Finally, the personal standards include their own safety mechanisms, which were neglected by the test subjects. These were trained by the test persons to avoid that not only the quality suffers due to forgetting or due to an error, but also that rework has to be done, which, depending on the extent, also leads to an increased feeling of stress afterwards. According to the participants, the mechanisms were triggered by carelessness, for example by reading the text carelessly. The reason was again time pressure. Thus, the personal safeguard against a later report by the committee in the supposedly upcoming meeting was no longer given, which created a feeling of fear and sometimes even panic in some subjects. In the interview, the subjects described the noncompliance with these safety mechanisms as a subjective feeling of stress.

3.2   Further Findings, Coping Strategies and Recommendations

Through the interviews, we were not only able to address the experiences of the work situation in the laboratory experiment. We also gained further insights regarding what happens in everyday work and about coping strategies for the right handling of stressful situations.

Frequent Interruptions and Coping. Participants also reported remote work experiences outside of the experiment. Thus, we could assume that frequent interruptions are more likely to use coping strategies that can be classified as problem-oriented coping according to the transactional stress model of Lazarus and Folkman [9]. According to their own statements, participants were aware of the interruptions each time and would work overtime on the same or another day to cope with the stress. Working on Saturdays was also reported as a possible solution, even if no contractual agreement existed. Alternatively, it was also reported that interruptions are simply no longer noticed after a certain point. This would occur if either the time required for the actual work was no longer sufficient and work content had to be completed at the same time or if effectiveness and efficiency were at risk. In such cases, the main task is given a higher priority and interruptions are rejected or not noticed. In addition, block appointments are used, which are entered in the calendar for superiors and colleagues. The business phone and messenger on the notebook are then also muted to achieve maximum isolation and avoid interruptions.

Recommendations for Stress Reduction. At the end of the interviews, all subjects were asked what advice they would give to a supervisor or manager after their experiences and the objective observation and discussion of their own job. Essentially, two main recommendations for avoiding stress emerged from the statements:

R1: Minimize or eliminate unnecessary interruptions through prioritization to ensure completion of major tasks at the employee's own discretion and to their own standards.
R2: Prioritize necessary interruptions/additional tasks, if possible, to those employees who have less work to do, to respect the concentrated work of busy employees.

Both require preliminary work by the manager or colleagues in the first instance. For example, the first step should be to check the calendar of the respective employee and, if necessary, ask about the time capacity. If a project has gone awry and a lot of time is needed by the people involved to work it through, their concentration should be respected. It would do the company, the manager, and the employee good to direct a potential interruption, if necessary, to the person who is currently available.

It is undisputed that even remote working cannot be completely uninterrupted without further measures. However, we assume that compliance with the above recommendations will already contribute to minimizing the employees' subjective sense of stress.

4   Limitations

This research examined, in a purely exploratory and qualitative manner, the effects of work interruptions in digital work and perceptions in terms of subjectively perceived stress. We used Lazarus and Folkman's transactional stress model (see Fig. 2) to classify the experiences from the experiment. Because physiological responses and effects do not necessarily correlate with psychological responses or subjective experience of stress [1], we limited this study to participants' sub-objective experiences.

4.1   Limitations of the Work Situation

We experimentally investigated the effects of interruptions in digital work under laboratory conditions. We decided against the experiment in the field to obtain results that are as comparable as possible. However, a work situation like the one we induced in the laboratory rarely occurs. We opted for interruptions by phone call and for additional tasks, which were writing a mail. But there are not only such disturbances.

We all know that push notifications on the business phone through all kinds of apps and messengers, notifications of incoming mails or messages, as well as calls via the communication medium used at work (e.g. Microsoft Teams, Skype for Business, etc.) can interrupt us in our work and keep us from doing it. It is the same with interruptions due to updates or failures in hardware and software. The possible disturbances caused by the job, or the devices and software required for it are manifold.

In addition, we can get interrupted in the home office also by our private environment: Construction noise on the street or in the same building, an ambulance driving by, or even our own children can keep us from working. Furthermore, the mailman, the neighbour, our pets as well as the house telephone can also be disruptive factors. Especially in interviews we found out that even our partner (who may not be able to work at home due to his job) can become a disturbance just by his presence and actions. Thus, many factors can interrupt the employee in his work outside the office. Accordingly, we assume that our findings regarding the stress experience in the field would have been significantly sharper depending on the individual disturbance.

4.2   Limitations Regarding the Experiment

Due to the increased effort, we decided to have two interruptions by call with additional tasks as well as another call without additional task in a period of 30 min. While other studies have conducted experiments lasting several hours [1,6] based on the original TSST [7] or TSST-related versions, our experiment is an exception. Furthermore, despite the choice of our work task, which we believe was inherently challenging but not impossible, we cannot rule out the possibility that simply the announced supposed presentation to a panel led to subjective feelings of stress. Although we asked the participants before the experiment whether they felt relaxed and fit and whether there was a tendency to stage fright or test anxiety, we cannot guarantee whether a tense basic attitude did not arise during the surprising announcement of the supposed presentation of the work results. In addition, we cannot exclude that during the experiment, for example, private messages led to a stress experience, because the subjects used their own notebooks as well as their own smartphones.

4.3   Limitations Regarding Comparability with the TSST

While various other studies used the TSST or a modified version of it, we decided to use a work situation as close to reality as possible, even under laboratory conditions. According to the original protocol of Kirschbaum et al. from 1993 [7], the TSST first includes a ten minute preparation time for an interview in front of a panel of managers, as well as its execution (with a duration of five minutes), during which a free speech is to be given. The participants are made to believe that the managers are specially trained to observe non-verbal behavior. In addition, tape recordings and a video analysis are to be made, which leads to the participants having the impression of being under constant observation. Furthermore, after a break, a serial subtraction task is to be performed in front of the panel, which also lasts five minutes. After each error, the subject must start again.

In our opinion, the TSST or a modified TSST version was rather less suitable for our research project. It is still important to consider that the TSST was used to provide demonstrably reliable physiological results [2], which was outside the scope of our research objective. Furthermore, we would like to point out again that the application of the TSST does not necessarily lead to a correlation of physiological stress and subjectively perceived stress [1]. Also the structure of the TSST's tasks is problematic regarding remote work. We tried to induce a work situation as close to reality as possible, which is based on a challenging work task, occupationally induced interruptions, and a supposed presentation of results. A serial subtraction task usually does not occur in remote work, nor does permanent observation, recording and analysis of non-verbal behavior by trained personnel.

Working remote is characterized by actual work and independent processing. In addition, there are meetings with and without webcam use, as well as interruptions induced by work and private life, which disturb employees in their work in various ways. From our point of view, our experiment is therefore less comparable to the use of the TSST, but it better represents the real situation from everyday life. So it was more suitable for our applied, explorative research approach.

5   Conclusion

As already mentioned, work interruptions are among the most important stressors in the workplace [13]. Therefore, they deserve special attention among other disturbing factors. In times of a changing world of work and the shift of work to the home office, we took the findings of the studies by Kerr et al. [6] and Campbell and Ehlert [1] as an opportunity to investigate the effects of work interruptions in digital working regarding the subjective perception of stress. Through our explorative and qualitative research approach, which was divided into a laboratory experiment with the use of eye-tracking as well as subsequent interviews, we were able to gain knowledge and formulate a hypothesis. The transactional stress model of Lazarus and Folkman from 1984 [9] was used to classify the stress experiences. It showed that disregarding personal standards at work leads to greater affective stress the greater the number of standards disregarded in remote work situations. This should be quantitatively verified in follow-up studies. In addition, we were able to gather further findings, for example on stress avoidance by supervisors and colleagues. For example, unnecessary interruptions should be minimized, or even eliminated, and necessary work interruptions should be directed to those employees who have the time capacity for them. In this way, concentrated employees will not be disturbed in their main tasks and their work will be respected. Overall, this research is a first step towards subjective stress research in digital work. Mental disorders are the second most common reason for work disability [11]. To prevent psychological disorders caused by stress and to reduce the resulting pathological consequences, future studies should continue to research these topics and develop approaches to avoid stress in digital work.

References

1. Campbell, J., Ehlert, U.: Acute psychosocial stress: does the emotional stress response correspond with physiological responses? Psychoneuroendocrinology **37**(8), 1111–1134 (2012)
2. Dickerson, S.S., Kemeny, M.E.: Acute stressors and cortisol responses: a theoretical integration and synthesis of laboratory research. Psychol. Bull. **130**(3), 355 (2004)
3. Emmler, H., Kohlrausch, B.: Homeoffice: Potenziale und Nutzung. Greenberger. Düsseldorf (WSI Policy Brief, 52) (2021)
4. Ernst, C.: Homeoffice im Kontext der Corona-Pandemie. Eine Ad-hoc-Studie der Technischen Hochschule Köln (2020)
5. Fertig, T., Henkelmann, D., Schütz, A.: 360 degrees of security: can VR increase the sustainability of ISA trainings? In: Proceedings of the 55th Hawaii International Conference on System Sciences (2022)
6. Kerr, J.I., et al.: The effects of acute work stress and appraisal on psychobiological stress responses in a group office environment. Psychoneuroendocrinology **121**, 104837 (2020)
7. Kirschbaum, C., Pirke, K.M., Hellhammer, D.H.: The 'Trier Social Stress Test'-a tool for investigating psychobiological stress responses in a laboratory setting. Neuropsychobiology **28**(1–2), 76–81 (1993)
8. Kuckartz, U., Rädiker, S.: Qualitative Inhaltsanalyse: Methoden, Praxis, Computerunterstützung: Grundlagentexte Methoden. Grundlagentexte Methoden, Beltz Juventa, Weinheim Basel, 5. auflage edn. (2022)
9. Lazarus, R.S., Folkman, S.: Stress, Appraisal and Coping. Springer Publishing Company, New York (1984). https://doi.org/10.1007/978-1-4419-1005-9_215

10. Misoch, S.: Qualitative Interviews. chap. 4.1 Das Leitfadeninterview, pp. 65–71. De Gruyter Oldenbourg (2015)
11. Statista: Wichtigste Krankheiten für Arbeitsunfähigkeit in Deutschland 2020. Technical report (2020). https://de.statista.com/statistik/daten/studie/250820/ umfrage/hauptkrankheitsarten-fuer-arbeitsunfaehigkeit-in-deutschland/
12. Ursin, H., Eriksen, H.R.: The cognitive activation theory of stress. Psychoneuroendocrinology **29**(5), 567–592 (2004)
13. Zapf, D., Semmer, N.K.: Stress und Gesundheit in Organisationen. Enzyklopädie der Psychologie, Themenbereich D, Serie **III**(3), 1007–1112 (2004)

COVID-19 Cases and Their Impact on Global Air Traffic

Regina Sousa[2(✉)]⬤, João Gomes[1], José Gomes[1], Mário Arcipreste[1],
Pedro Guimarães[1], Daniela Oliveira[2]⬤, and José Machado[2]⬤

[1] University of Minho, Braga, Portugal
{PG47306,PG47367,PG47501,PG47582}@alunos.uminho.pt
[2] ALGORITMI/LASI, University of Minho, Braga, Portugal
{regina.sousa,daniela.oliveira}@algoritmi.uminho.pt, jmac@di.uminho.pt

Abstract. The air transport industry has marked unprecedented changes throughout the pandemic period of Covid-19 infection. Mostly in the number of flights canceled, liquidation of airlines and disconnection between points worldwide. The existing documentation relating to air traffic, in the specific period of this study, can be extracted, processed and visualized through tools widely used to support case study assumptions, especially in the context of Big Data. This document addresses to the use of a Big Data architecture to survey, analyze and explore different data sources and consequent loading, transformation and visual representation of the results obtained in order to verify the impact of the number of cases of infection by Covid-19 in air traffic. Based on the results obtained through the described methodology, it can be stated that the number of cases of infection by Covid-19 presents a significant impact on the number of flights that occurred ever since (around 50% less flights).

Keywords: Covid-19 World Impact · GDP · Big Data Architecture · Air Traffic

1 Introduction and Motivation

The World Health Organization declared the existence of a global SARS-CoV-2 pandemic in the first months of 2020, since then revealing itself as a challenge in the most diverse aspects [9]. Therefore, one of the most affected sectors corresponds to air transport, in which there were heavy restrictions in terms of the different categories of flights and, consequently, significant losses in financial matters. In this sense, it is particularly relevant to infer how and to what extent the number of cases of Covid-19 infection contributed to the setback seen in the air transport industry, in particular in the number of flights performed. This process can be carried out through the analysis of data sources to support the case study, based on the use of tools for this purpose [10].

The current context presents a wide range of tools for extracting, transforming and visualizing data at different levels of use, more geared towards certain

ICST Institute for Computer Sciences, Social Informatics and Telecommunications Engineering 2023
Published by Springer Nature Switzerland AG 2023. All Rights Reserved
J. M. Machado and H. Peixoto (Eds.): AISCOVID 2022, LNICST 485, pp. 16–27, 2023.
https://doi.org/10.1007/978-3-031-38204-8_2

circumstances to the detriment of others [4]. Even so, their common purpose is endowed with significant relevance to the context of data analysis, Big Data and statistics, and, consequently, to the case study in question.

This article is structured in four sections: related work, for gathering information on previously carried out researches and publications that follow the same or somewhat similar case studies; materials and methods, where are specified data sources, Big Data architecture to support the case study, as well as the work environment in which the study takes place and the approaches considered throughout the loading, processing and transformation processes and visual representation of the results; results, for the presentation of the information obtained through the application of the aforementioned processes; and a section for discussing the results, where the data obtained in the context of the case study is critically portrayed and an attempt is made to identify possible improvements with the objective of enriching its value.

2 Related Work

In order to compare and analyse our future results, we started by searching for previous assignments around the same subject of study. Hence, in this section, we will approach how these themes are connected to our purpose, explaining and comparing the results collected with the ones we are expecting to obtain throughout our analysis.

2.1 Impact of Coronavirus (COVID-19) Pandemic on Air Transport Mobility, Energy, and Environment: A Case Study [1]

Firstly, this is a straight example of a project that follows the same ideologies as ours although it includes a more specific approach to the theme since the analysis is made to two airports in particular, in Croatia. This condition may lead to a different set of results compared to the ones we may get because we are working with much more general type of data. Furthermore, they also have side observations such as the study of the CO_2 levels alongside the number of flights in a certain airport and the analysis of the cargo flights component.

Nonetheless, it is possible to infer that the conclusions present in this project may be similar to ours since it's almost obvious that the number of flights decreased due to the pandemic situation. As mentioned above, our results may very in terms of percentage values since our case of study applies to many different countries, leading to a different set of results and conclusions.

2.2 Estimating and Projecting Air Passenger Traffic During the COVID-19 Coronavirus Outbreak and Its Socio-Economic Impact [2]

In contrast to our analysis, where we will seek to investigate the impact of Covid-19 on the airline industry for the last few years, this study from 2020 aimed to estimate the effects of air travel ban on aviation and its socio-economic impact for the following years based on historical data from January 2010 till October 2019. Therefore, a forecasting model, which made use of airplane movements extracted from online flight tracking platforms and on-line booking systems, was implemented in order to set a reference baseline,

As a result, it turned out that, according to these hypothetical scenarios, in the first Quarter of 2020 the impact of aviation losses could have negatively reduced World GDP by 0.02% to 0.12% according to the observed data and, in the worst case scenarios, at the end of 2020 the loss could be as high as 1.41–1.67% and job losses may reach the value of 25–30 millions. Focusing on EU27, the GDP loss may amount to 1.66–1.98% by the end of 2020 and the number of job losses from 4.2 to 5 millions in the worst case scenarios.

By the end of the current study, we will be able to carry out a comparative analysis between the estimated results with the results actually obtained for the evolution of GDP in the year 2020.

2.3   Global Impact of COVID-19 Pandemic on Road Traffic Collisions [3]

Similarly to our project, this example aims to review the impact of COVID-19 on a certain area, but in contrast, instead of analysing the effect of this virus on the world air traffic, it focuses on the incidence, patterns, and severity of the injury, management, and outcomes of RTCs and give recommendations on improving road safety during the pandemic. All the data used in this given project was extracted from many RTCs published in English language using PubMed, Scopus and Google Scholar, as well as Google search engine and websites to retrieve relevant published literature, including discussion papers, reports, and media news.

The results obtained in the end conclude that traffic volume dropped during the COVID-19 pandemic which was associated with significant drop in RTCs globally and a reduction of road deaths in 32 out of 36 countries in April 2020 compared with April 2019. There was also a decrease in annual road death in 33 out of 42 countries in 2020 compared with 2019. The opposite occurred in four and nine countries during the periods, respectively. There was also a drop in the number of admitted patients in trauma centers related to RTCs during both periods. This has been attributed to an increase in speeding, emptier traffic lanes, reduced law enforcement, not wearing seat belts, alcohol and drug abuse.

Despite the fact that different percentages may be obtained, since the case study and the sample are distinct, it is expected that the results from our project may follow a similar route, in terms of traffic volume, since many measures were applied to the airports, in order to reduce the spread of COVID-19.

3   Materials and Methods

The shown architecture in Fig. 1 comprises a consistent pipeline of data storage, processing, and analysis, assuming a strong influence of the Apache ecosystem, specifically the Hadoop system, and supporting the case study evaluation based on the collected datasets.

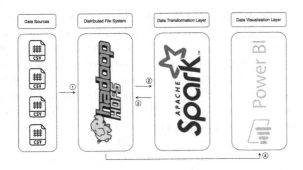

Fig. 1. Proposed Big Data architecture

It was possible to design an ecosystem to support data processing and visualisation to answer the case study, producing a Big Data architecture, based on the set of tools available for designing analysis-oriented architectures for Big Data systems, as well as their respective advantages and disadvantages.

A three-layer system is proposed to evaluate the influence of the number of SARS-CoV-2 infection cases on aviation traffic. The first element of the architecture represents the selection of data sources that communicate with the distributed file system, which is in charge of connecting and storing the supplied data. Despite sharing foundations with the GlusterFS tool, for example, Hadoop HDFS is preferable to the alternative because it allows for simpler integration with Apache ecosystem products and performs better for activities conducted close to the data.

The data is then sent to the processing layer through the Apache Spark tool, which does concurrent, distributed analysis. For the purposes of this study, the Spark tool is chosen over Apache Kafka because it supports native Extract, Transform, and Load (ETL) services and the usage of a micro-batch processing strategy, which is superior to an event-driven continuous processing model.

Finally, the end result of the data processing may be queried using the Microsoft Power BI tool, which retrieves the relevant data directly from the Hadoop tool's HDFS. Tableau is a reasonable solution for this purpose, but it comes with costs associated with its use, as well as less mobility in terms of analysis and representation alternatives accessible.

3.1   Data Sources

The data sources selected for the present research focus on four main themes: COVID-19 infection status, flights taken, population status, and Gross Domestic Product (GDP). Only one dataset is considered for each of the first, third, and fourth themes mentioned above, while the second theme falls into three datasets.

For the above-mentioned datasets, the corresponding annotation period runs from 2020 to May 2022 and is spread out by country.

Daily Infections by Covid-19 (WHO). The first dataset considered reports official World Health Organization (WHO) data regarding the daily number of Covid-19 infections and deaths over the course of vaccine administration reported by different countries and territories. This data source is particularly relevant because of its direct relationship to the case study, and secondly because of the legitimacy and international recognition of the organization providing it, in addition to presenting figures on a daily basis [5]. This dataset consists of 8 columns characterized as follows: Date of reporting to WHO; ISO Alpha-2 country code; Country, territory, area; WHO regional offices; New confirmed cases. Calculated by subtracting previous cumulative case count from current cumulative cases count; Cumulative confirmed cases reported to WHO to date; New confirmed deaths. Calculated by subtracting previous cumulative deaths from current cumulative deaths; Cumulative confirmed deaths reported to WHO to date.

Daily Flights Performed. The air traffic dataset reports the daily data obtained regarding the number of flights performed in different countries and territories in a given year. Like the last one, this source is good for analysis because it has a direct link to the case study and gives daily data, which makes it easy to compare with data from the previous year [6].

The daily flights performed dataset from 2020 consists of 9 columns, characterised as follows: Name of the State; ISO week of 'Day'; Day of the year (YYYY-MM-DD format); Number of flights for 'Entity' on 'Day'; 7-day moving average of number of flights on 'Day'; Reference date in 2019 with respect to 'Day'; Number of flights for 'Entity' on 'Day 2019'; Percentage change in number of flights on 'Day' compared to 'Day 2019'; 7-day moving average percentage change in number of flights on 'Day' with respect to 'Day 2019'.

The daily flights performed in datasets from 2021 and 2022 consist of two additional columns compared to the previous one. These columns are characterised as follows: Reference date in the previous year with respect to 'Day'; Number of flights on 'Day Previous Year'.

Population. The dataset associated with this theme includes statistics for the current population as reported by different countries and territories, counting all residents regardless of their citizenship. This data source reveals some applicability in this matter, as it allows for verifying the existence - or absence - of relationships between the existing population and the two main components of the case study [7].

The population status dataset consists of 65 columns characterized as follows: Country, territory, area; ISO Alpha-2 country code; World Development Indicator name; World Development Indicator code; Population numbers of each year between 1960 to 2021.

Gross Domestic Product (GDP). The dataset that falls on this topic includes statistics for the GDP indicator as reported by different countries and territories. This data source applies for some applicability to the case study as it allows for verifying the existence - or absence - of any relationship between the fluctuation of GDP and the two main components of the case study [8]. This dataset also consists of 65 columns equally characterized as the previous data source.

3.2 Data Transformation Layer

Aviation and COVID-19 situations require the greatest processing. For the first datasets, the main approach focuses on selecting the most relevant columns, including the number of flights performed daily and according to 7-day travel periods, the number of flights performed for the previous year, and the chronological reference of these records for 2020, 2021, and 2022. 2020 data allows 2019 data. For each dataset, removing the year from the date item in the column names is examined. This index repair process consolidates theme-related material.

After this approach, the nations that intersect the newly formed dataset and COVID-19 are determined, resulting in a filtering process on both datasets. This method removes unnecessary columns from the second-most-relevant dataset. To obtain a processed dataset comparable to the number of flights, the dataset under investigation is partitioned into 3 new datasets, one for each year, with the respective identification in the related columns. This component's data sets are integrated using a similar method.

For datasets with a lot of 1960–2020 columns, most columns are eliminated and only the nation and year columns are picked and filtered. Finally, the data are consolidated into one daily row per country. Each country has 365 rows since years are columnar.

Next, seven main references whose analysis is pertinent to the case study and the resulting dataset were found. Seven references are:

1. Number of registered Covid-19 cases by country;
2. Total number of Covid-19 cases registered;
3. Number of flights performed by country;
4. Total number of cases of flights performed;
5. Value of GDP obtained by country;
6. Difference between the GDP values obtained by country;
7. Total number of registered Covid-19 cases and flights carried out.

According to the previous enumeration, each reference selected for analysis should be saved in Comma-Separated Values format files. This approach reduces the work necessary for data selection and visual reproduction to facilitate data imports into a visualisation tool. For 1., 3., and 5., the methodology is based on selecting the necessary set of columns from the pre-processed data dataset. Following a similar process in the previous instance, 2. and 4. introduce a sum feature. In example 6, the 2019 GDP figures are subtracted from the 2020 GDP values. In case 7, the smaller datasets from cases 2. and 4. are joined with a modest orientation change to improve graphical display.

3.3   Data Visualization Layer

The visualisation component considers importing Hadoop HDFS results by connecting to its address. For each of the previous section's important points, the appropriate processed dataset is loaded in Comma-separated values format and presented according to several sorts of views and graphic elements, with particular emphasis on bar graphs.

4   Results

Through transformation procedures, a dataset that meets the investigation's essential points was obtained. The same dataset was then shown using Microsoft Power BI. Figure 3 compares new Covid-19 cases by nation in 2020 and 2021. Figure 3 shows the difference in total cases between 2020 and 2021.

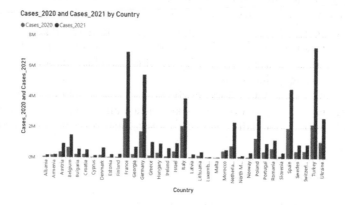

Fig. 2. Number of registered Covid-19 cases by country in 2020 and 2021.

Figures 2 and 3 show that the number of new cases of infection increased significantly in 2020 to 20 million, while more than doubling in 2021, with 51 million cases, representing nearly 73% of the total cases seen in the two-year aggregate. These statistics are especially noticeable in larger countries like France, Germany, Italy, Spain, and Turkey, which serve as air traffic hubs.

In terms of the analysis of the number of flights performed in the countries in question, the following figures were obtained, in which the first graph represents the number of flights performed in the years 2019, 2020 and 2021 - Fig. 4, while the second graph demonstrates the difference of the number of flights performed, as a percentage of the total, in the years 2019, 2020 and 2021 - Fig. 5:

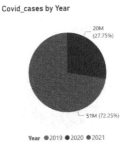

Covid_cases by Year

Year ● 2019 ● 2020 ● 2021

Fig. 3. Total number of Covid-19 cases registered in 2020 and 2021.

Figure 4 shows France, Germany, Italy, Spain, and Turkey have more flights. This picture shows a 50% drop in flights between 2019 and 2020. 2020 and 2021 show a small increase. Figure 5 illustrates the consolidation of all the numbers for the sample nations, revealing that of all the flights between 2019 and 2021, almost 50% took place in the first year, with 2020 comprising just around 22% of all flights. Flights will increase from 6 million in 2020 to 8 million in 2021. After analysing the countries' confirmed GDP, the following results were found: Figs. 6 and 7 show 2019 and 2020 GDP and their difference.

Similarly to the two previous cases, the values for the GDP for the six countries, between the years of 2019 and 2020, show a generalized decline, with a special impact on the aforementioned countries, particularly France, Italy and Spain, which show a reduction around 100 to 150 billion dollars as seen in Figs. 6 and 7. This decrease makes sense in light of the need to paralyze some economic sectors, of which the air transport sector represents an important component, due to the number of cases verified for the respective years. Even so, this com-

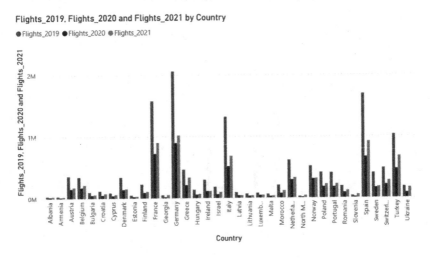

Flights_2019, Flights_2020 and Flights_2021 by Country

● Flights_2019 ● Flights_2020 ● Flights_2021

Fig. 4. Number of flights performed by country in 2019, 2020 and 2021.

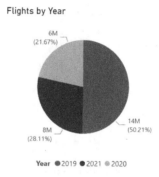

Fig. 5. Total number of flight cases performed in 2019, 2020 and 2021.

ponent cannot be weighted with the same proportion compared to the previous components, since it concerns a smaller sample, taking into account the absence of GDP values for the year of 2021. In fact, this aspect of the case of study can be improved in terms of the information transmitted through the integration, when available, of data for the mentioned year.

Finally, with regard to the intersection of the data obtained for the number of cases of Covid-19 and for the number of flights performed, in the years of 2019, 2020 and 2021, the following graph was obtained, in which the bars represent the first component and the line represents the second component, respectively:

Finally, in order to obtain information from the intersection between the main components of the study, namely the number of cases of infection by Covid-19 and the number of flights carried out in the years of 2019, 2020 and 2021, there is Fig. 8. According to the analysis already carried out, the number of cases of Covid-19 infection increases from year to year, while the number of flights performed decreases at an early stage and recovers slightly in the last year.

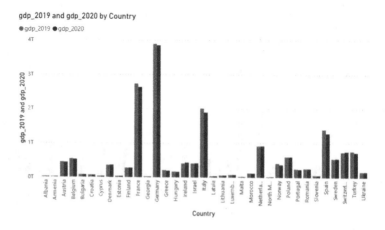

Fig. 6. GDP value obtained by country in 2019 and 2020.

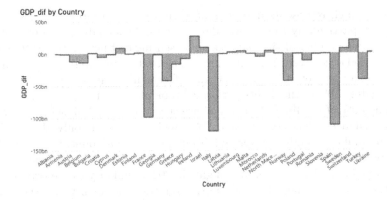

Fig. 7. Difference between the GDP values obtained by country in 2019 and 2020.

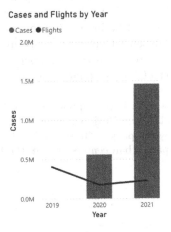

Fig. 8. Total number of registered Covid-19 cases and performed flights in 2019, 2020 and 2021.

With these data, there is a relatively peculiar condition regarding the year of 2021.

As can be seen, the nature of the case study takes particular advantage of visual references supported by bar graphs or similar graphs.

5   Conclusions and Future Work

The air transport industry suffered unprecedented changes over the Covid-19 pandemic period, in particular relatively to the number of flights canceled, airline liquidation and disconnection between points worldwide. One of the main methods to evaluate the existence of correlations between the circumstances of this phenomenon is based on the use of analytics associated with the concept of

Big Data, which represents data sets of great variety, in large volumes and at high speed, particularly from newer data sources. This analysis is supported by a considerable number of Big Data tools, presenting distinct characteristics with equally varied objectives, from data processing to its intuitive representation. To summarize, for the set of countries (France, Germany, Italy, Spain, and Turkey), approximately 50% of the flights performed took place in the first year, while the remaining 50% of the flights performed are spread over the following two years, with particular emphasis on the year 2020, which represents only about 22% of the total number of flights performed. Taking this into account, it is possible to see, as previously stated, a slight recovery in these terms, with an increase from 6 million flights in 2020 to 8 million flights in 2021. Similarly to the two previous cases, the values for the GDP for the six countries, between the years of 2019 and 2020, show a generalized decline, with a special impact on the aforementioned countries, particularly France, Italy and Spain, which show a reduction around 100 to 150 billion dollars. For a better assessment of the impact caused over the 2 stated years, it would be interesting to consider the values for 2022. As mentioned above, the present study takes place in June 2022, which means the existing data for the different existing components do not reflect the same sample necessary for a correct and adequate comparison.

Aknowledgements. This work has been supported by FCT—Fundação para a Ciência e Tecnologia within the R&D Units Project Scope: UIDB/00319/2020. The grant of Regina Sousa is supported by the project "Integrated and Innovative Solutions for the well-being of people in complex urban centers" within the Project Scope NORTE-01-0145-FEDER-000086.

References

1. Nižetić, S.: Impact of coronavirus (covid-19) pandemic on air transport mobility, energy, and environment: a case study. Int. J. Energy Res. **44**(13), 10953–10961 (2020)
2. Iacus, S.M., Natale, F., Santamaria, C., Spyratos, S., Vespe, M.: Estimating and projecting air passenger traffic during the COVID-19 coronavirus outbreak and its socio-economic impact. Saf. Sci. **129**, 104791 (2020)
3. Yasin, Y.J., Grivna, M., Abu-Zidan, F.M.: Global impact of COVID-19 pandemic on road traffic collisions. World J. Emerg. Surg. **16**(1), 1–14 (2021)
4. Sousa, R., Miranda, R., Moreira, A., Alves, C., Lori, N., Machado, J.: Software tools for conducting real-time information processing and visualization in industry: an up-to-date review. Appl. Sci. **11**(11), 4800 (2021)
5. WHO COVID-19 Dashboard. Geneva: World Health Organization (2020). https://covid19.who.int/
6. Eurocontrol Dashboard: Daily Traffic Variation - States (2020). https://www.eurocontrol.int/Economics/DailyTrafficVariation-States.html
7. The World Bank Dashboard: Population, total (2019). https://data.worldbank.org/indicator/SP.POP.TOTL
8. The World Bank Dashboard: GPD (US$) (2020). https://data.worldbank.org/indicator/NY.GDP.MKTP.CD

9. Oliveira, D., et al.: Management of a pandemic based on an openehr approach. Proc. Comput. Sci. **177**, 522–527 (2020)
10. Hak, F., Guimarães, T., Abelha, A., Santos, M.: An exploratory study of a NoSQL database for a clinical data repository. In: Rocha, Á., Adeli, H., Reis, L.P., Costanzo, S., Orovic, I., Moreira, F. (eds.) WorldCIST 2020. AISC, vol. 1161, pp. 476–483. Springer, Cham (2020). https://doi.org/10.1007/978-3-030-45697-9_46

The Impact of Contingency Measures on the COVID-19 Reproduction Rate

Regina Sousa🆔, Daniela Oliveira🆔, Francini Hak🆔, and José Machado$^{(\boxtimes)}$🆔

ALGORITMI/LASI, University of Minho, Braga, Portugal
{regina.sousa,daniela.oliveira,francini.hak}@algoritmi.uminho.pt,
jmac@di.uminho.pt

Abstract. The SARS-CoV-2 virus had a major impact on the health of the world's population, causing governments to take progressively more cautious measures. All of these measures took into account the pandemic situation in the region in real time, with the aim of slowing down the spread of the infection as much as possible and reducing the associated mortality. This article aims to study the impact of preventive measures on the spread of COVID-19 and the consequent impact on excess deaths. In order to obtain the results presented, Big Data techniques were used for data storage and processing. As a result it can be concluded that Gross Domestic Product (GDP) is directly proportional to the Human Development Index (HDI), Higher GDP per capita are associated with a higher number of new cases of COVID-19 and R-index is inversely proportional to the severity of the contingency measures.

Keywords: Covid-19 · Contigency Measures · Proliferation rate · Correlation · Big Data Analysis · Spark · PowerBI

1 Introduction

In March 2020, the World Health Organization (WHO) declared a worldwide pandemic derived from the new class of Coranavirus. Contingency measures were adopted, changing face-to-face activities to a virtual format, depriving some habits, closing local businesses and forcing people to confine themselves at home for months [4]. Being a novelty, no country knew how to properly deal with the pandemic and which measures would be most effective, always taking into account other concerns, such as the country's economy and people's mental health [7].

A consequence of the pandemic was the daily production of data, that grew exponentially. Big Data techniques were applied to treat and analyze the data in the proper way, in order to generate knowledge to support decision-making processes [11]. Thus, it was possible to monitor in real time the evolution of cases of infection and deaths caused in each country [5]. In this sense, this article aims to apply Big Data techniques to verify whether or not the contingency measures contributed to reducing the spread of the Covid-19 virus.

ICST Institute for Computer Sciences, Social Informatics and Telecommunications Engineering 2023
Published by Springer Nature Switzerland AG 2023. All Rights Reserved
J. M. Machado and H. Peixoto (Eds.): AISCOVID 2022, LNICST 485, pp. 28–37, 2023.
https://doi.org/10.1007/978-3-031-38204-8_3

The paper is divided into five sections. First, an introduction is made in which the reader is informed about the theme and purpose of the document. The second section provides context for the topic discussed. Following that, the study's materials and methods are described. The results are presented in Sect. 4. Finally, conclusions are reached, as well as next steps for future work.

2 Background

With the accelerating adoption of Information Technologies (IT), the amount of data produced daily has been increasing exponentially [12]. Traditional data storage and management processes are no longer enough. In this sense, the term Big Data emerged, capable of extracting, processing and analyzing large amounts of data in real time, dealing with complex and different data structures [10].

Big Data is characterized by 5 Vs, such as: (i) volume in relation to the amount of data collected; (ii) velocity defined by the time of processing and manipulation of the data; (iii) variety of acquired data types; (iv) veracity to the quality, reliability and accuracy of the data provided; (v) value obtained with the collected data [10].

Data analysis is recognized by the ability to transform raw data into knowledge, in order to support the decision-making. This process is usually divided into three phases: Storage, Processing and Visualization [12]. As such, there are several tools destined to each phase of the process, however, some can run more than one phase. Some commonly used tools in the storage phase are MongoDB, Apache Cassandra and CouchDB. For the processing phase there are tools like Apache Spark, Apache Hadoop and Samza. For the last phase we can find tools such as PowerBI, Tableau and Stat iQ.

Big data has proven to be essential in the healthcare sector, being able to handle a huge amount of data to provide real-time monitoring of epidemic outbreaks [2]. In relation to previous outbreaks of epidemics and pandemics, COVID-19 is unprecedented, so it was necessary that datasets be created and made available as open access, for possible analysis of the daily numbers of new infections broken down by country or cities [4]. Thus, computational techniques allowed us to visualize the spread of the virus in real time, have an accurate detection of infected patients, and obtain an optimized contact tracing. However, there are still points that need to be analyzed and this article aims to analyze whether the application of contingency measures in fact contributed to reducing the spread of Covid-19.

3 Materials and Methods

The main goal of this research work is to study the impact that imposed containment measures have had on the proliferation rate of COVID-19 infection, worldwide. To do this, public datasets were used with data on the rates of measures applied in different geographic areas over time, as well as data on COVID-19 indicators in each region and their reproduction rate. According to the defined case study, the following research question emerged, which this work aims to answer:

How did government measures during COVID-19 affect the reproduction rate?

3.1 Big Data Architecture

Given the high amount of data for processing, it was necessary to develop an architecture subdivided by four distinct phases, the first being the choice and fusion of the various data sources, whose output will be the input of the next phase, called Storage. The processed data will then go through the central phase of the research, which is the data processing and its respective treatment using the Apache Spark tool. In order to be able to draw conclusions and construct some Business Intelligence indicators, the Visualization phase was planned, using the PowerBI tool. The architecture present in the Fig. 1 meticulously demonstrates all the processes.

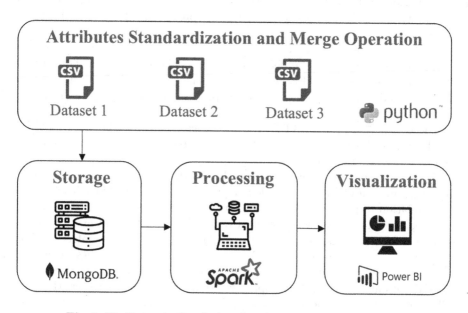

Fig. 1. Big Data pipeline designed and its phases implemented.

Data Collection and Storage: To answer the case study correctly, 3 public datasets were chosen and will be presented below. All datasets are in CSV format although with different time horizons.

- **First Dataset - WHO COVID-19 Global Data:** The WHO COVID-19 Global Data dataset contains information associated with the COVID-19 pandemic in each of 236 countries from January 3, 2020, to March 1, 2022. It consists of 8 attributes that serve as the basis for subsequent datasets, with information such as the number of new COVID-19 cases per day and cumulative, and the number of COVID-19 deaths per day, for each country, its code, and its respective region for the World Health Organization (WHO) [8].

- **Second Dataset - COVID-19 Government Response Tracker:** This dataset consists of 6 attributes that are intended to represent the degree of severity associated with the government measures imposed in each country. Each observed country is associated with its daily percentage index of health and confinement for exposure, called **Containment Health Index For Display**, and its health and confinement index designated on a scale of 0 to 3. The time horizon for this dataset starts on January 1, 2020 and ends on February 3, 2021 [3].

- **Third Dataset - COVID-19 by *Our World in Data*:** This information source is composed of 67 attributes referring to different indicators evaluated against the impact of COVID-19, such as confirmed cases and deaths, excess mortality, hospital and ICU occupation, policy responses, tests and positivity, vaccinations, and reproduction rate. In this case study, special attention was given to the **Reproduction Rate** (**R** indicator) indicator, which estimates in real time the effective reproduction rate of COVID-19. The **Location** and **Date** attributes were also necessary to be able to join with the other datasets chosen [1].

- **Final Dataset Acquisition:** To get to the final dataset, the three data sets described above were joined using a script developed in Python using the Pandas library. This library is one of the most used today for the treatment of data with different types of data, allowing simple and effective manipulation [9]. The merge operation of the different datasets was done through the attributes **Location** and **Date**, which are present in both. To do this, it was necessary to first rename these two attributes in all the datasets so that they had the same designation. Additionally, it was necessary to format all dates in the *yyyy-mm-dd* format. Lastly, the final dataset obtained is uploaded into a Mongo database.

Data Processing: An Extraction, Transformation, and Loading (ETL) process was developed, where data stored in the Mongo database was obtained (*Extract*) to be properly treated (*Transformation*). Using the PySpark library, the transformation of this data was performed. Finally, the resulting data was saved in a Databricks table to be able to be queried by a data visualization platform (*Loading*). The data processing phase was subdivided into the following tasks:

- **Redundant columns removal:** After an analysis of the dataset, the removal of some redundant and duplicate columns that had no relevance to the case study was performed;

- **Removal of new negative COVID-19 case records:** Removal of records with negative new COVID-19 cases: Records whose number of new daily COVID-19 cases had a negative value were removed;

- **Removal of R indicator null values:** For the primary purpose of analyzing the R indicator, records with a reproduction rate of null have been removed.

Data Visualization: Data visualization is the last stage of the proposed architecture, ending with the graphical representation of information and the creation of dashboards to analyze the impact of government measures on the COVID-19 reproduction rate. The tool chosen for information visualization was PowerBI and allows connection to other data sources such as Spark and Azure Databricks [6]. A connection was made to the cluster created on the Databricks platform to query the data resulting from the processing step described above.

4   Results

Taking into account the previously described architecture, all the preprocessing and data manipulation culminated in dashboards, built in PowerBI. Therefore, some of the components of the final dashboard will be analyzed and discussed in the following section. Initially, bar charts were generated (one to verify the gross domestic product (GDP) per capita by location and another for the human development index also by location).

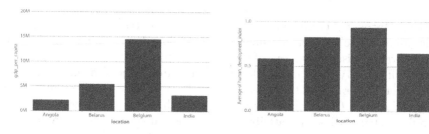

(a) Gross domestic product per capita per location.

(b) Human development index per location.

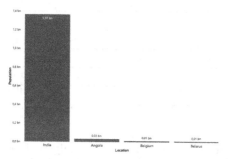

(c) Number of Population per location.

Fig. 2. Initial feature analysis.

Analyzing the results, the Fig. 2a shows the 4 selected countries. This selection was made taking into account its representativeness, presenting two countries with a low per capita GDP (Angola and India), a country with a medium GDP value (Belarus) and a country with a high GDP value (Belgium). It should also be noted that two countries with low GDP per capita were selected so that it was possible to relate the amount of population to the remaining parameters, considering for Angola a population of 32 million [13] and for India of 1.3 billion [14]. The Fig. 2b shows the relations between the human development index by country, confirming that although all of them have relatively high rates, Angola and India are a little below average.

On the other hand, the Fig. 3 represents the evolution of the virus proliferation rate (R) for each country, in the time interval of the collected data. Through its analysis, it can be concluded that countries with higher values for the R indicator also have a higher Gross Domestic Product (GDP) per capita and a higher human development index, which may also be related to the fact that their populations are older. However, the R-indicator of India, which has a significantly lower GDP per capita, is also high due to the fact that this country maintains a high containment health index when compared to the number of new COVID-19 cases, this correlation can be analyzed in Fig. 3 and Fig. 4.

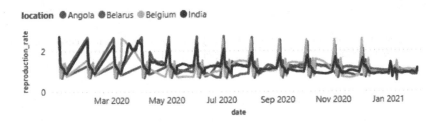

Fig. 3. Virus proliferation rate, over time.

Now presenting the correlations between various parameters, the relationship between Containment Health For Display (severity of containment measures) and the percentage of new cases per country is illustrated in Fig. 4. In this figure it can be concluded that the rate of contingency measures in most countries is directly proportional to the average number of cases. Only in India, the rate of contingency measures is higher than the number of cases, which is justified by the Fig. 3, where it is shown that the number of cases decreased probably due to the level of restrictions imposed over a long period of time.

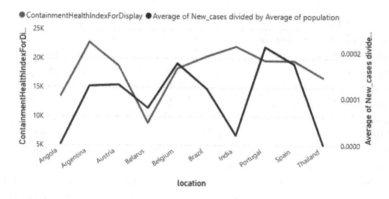

Fig. 4. Evolution of severity of contingency measures with the number of new cases, per location.

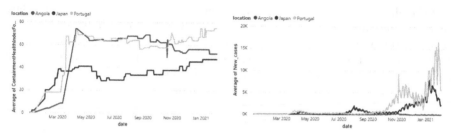

(a) Average Contingency Measure Index over time per location.

(b) Average number of new cases over time per location.

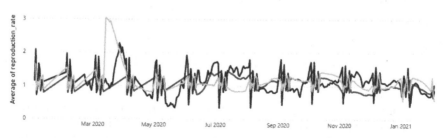

(c) Variance of the average virus proliferation rate over time per location.

Fig. 5. Comparative analysis between the means of the contingency measures, number of new infection cases COVID-19 and R-indicator.

A detailed analysis of the graphs presented in Fig. 5a, Fig. 5b and Fig. 5c shows that the containment measures emerged in response to the high probability of infection (proliferation rate).

An example is Portugal where, when the reproduction rate and new cases rose sharply, the severity of the containment measures increased considerably. Here, too, we can see that the containment measures affect the reproduction rate, because when the measures were kept at a high level, the proliferation rate was somewhat contained.

Moreover, comparing Japan and Portugal, the higher value of the reproduction rate of the former is about half of the latter, this is due to the fact that Japan implemented containment measures before Portugal, and thus the probability of infection was much lower.

Overall, analyzing the Fig. 6, it can be seen that the containment measures emerged in response to a high proliferation rate. It is further concluded that stabilization of the containment measures at high levels provided stabilization of the proliferation rate at relatively low levels.

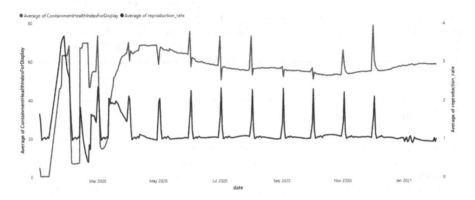

Fig. 6. Overall assessment of the average of the containment measures against the average of the R-indicator.

5   Conclusions and Future Work

A Big Data architecture was developed with emerging technologies in the market, such as Apache Spark, Azure Databricks, NoSQL databases such as MongoDB, and PowerBI, with the purpose of analyzing the impact of government measures against the proliferation rate of COVID-19.

The GDP was analyzed in relation to the population of each country and its Human Development Index (HDI). It was found that the GDP is directly proportional to the HDI, as opposed to the value of each country's population, as is the case of Angola and India. It was also concluded that countries with a higher GDP per capita are associated with a higher number of new cases of COVID-19, which is related to the existence of better access to health care and, consequently, a higher number of tests performed. Another premise is that air transport is also more abundant in these countries, so the COVID-19 contamination of travelers is directly proportional.

The severity index of contingency measures applied in each country was found to increase in the face of high R-indicator values and high numbers of new cases of COVID-19 infection. The R-indicator is therefore inversely proportional to the severity of the contingency measures.

Therefore, it can be concluded that the application of contingency measures influenced the pandemic situation in each country differently. There are countries that used contingency measures as prevention, and in these cases a decrease in the number of cases is more effective.

On the other side, there are countries that used contingency measures as a response to the increase in the number of cases. In this last scenario the control of the pandemic was not as effective. The graphs that best illustrate this phenomenon are shown in Figs. 5a, 5b and 5c.

Acknowledgements. This work has been supported by FCT-Fundação para a Ciência e Tecnologia within the R&D Units Project Scope: UIDB/00319/2020. The grant of Regina Sousa is supported by the project "Integrated and Innovative Solutions for the well-being of people in complex urban centers" within the Project Scope NORTE-01-0145-FEDER-000086. Francini Hak thanks the Fundação para a Tecnologia (FCT) for the grant 2021.06230.BD.

References

1. Appel, C., et al.: Data on covid-19 (coronavirus) by our world in data. https://github.com/owid/covid-19-data/tree/master/public/data. Accessed 01 May 05 2022
2. Bragazzi, N.L., Dai, H., Damiani, G., Behzadifar, M., Martini, M., Wu, J.: How big data and artificial intelligence can help better manage the covid-19 pandemic. Int. J. Environ. Res. Public Health **17** (2020). https://doi.org/10.3390/ijerph17093176
3. of Government, B.S.: Oxford covid-19 government response tracker. https://static-content.springer.com/esmart%3A10.1038%2Fs41562-021-01079-8/MediaObjects/41562_2021_1079_MOESM4_ESM.xlsx. Accessed 01 May 05 2022
4. Hak, F., Abelha, A., Santos, M.: Open science in pandemic times: a literature review. vol. 177, pp. 552–555. Elsevier B.V. (2020). https://doi.org/10.1016/j.procs.2020.10.077
5. Leung, C.K., Chen, Y., Shang, S., Deng, D.: Big data science on covid-19 data, pp. 14–21. Institute of Electrical and Electronics Engineers Inc., December 2020. https://doi.org/10.1109/BigDataSE50710.2020.00010
6. Microsoft: Tutorial: Introdução ao serviço de criação no power bi. microsoft documentation. https://docs.microsoft.com/pt-pt/power-bi/fundamentals/service-get-started, July 2020, Accessed 16 May 2022
7. Oliveira, D., et al.: Management of a pandemic based on an openehr approach. Procedia Comput. Sci. **177**, 522–527 (2020)
8. Organization, W.H.: Who coronavirus (covid-19) dashboard — who coronavirus (covid-19) dashboard with vaccination data. https://covid19.who.int/data, Accessed 01 May 2022
9. Pandas: Pandas - python data analysis library. https://pandas.pydata.org/, Accessed 01 May 2022
10. Sagiroglu, S., Sinanc, D.: Big data: a review, pp. 42–47 (2013). https://doi.org/10.1109/CTS.2013.6567202

11. Sousa, R., Lima, T., Abelha, A., Machado, J.: Hierarchical temporal memory theory approach to stock market time series forecasting. Electronics **10**(14), 1630 (2021)
12. Tsai, C.-W., Lai, C.-F., Chao, H.-C., Vasilakos, A.V.: Big data analytics: a survey. J. Big Data **2**(1), 1–32 (2015). https://doi.org/10.1186/s40537-015-0030-3
13. Worldometer: angola population live (2022). https://www.worldometers.info/world-population/angola-population/. Accessed 16 May 2022
14. Worldometer: India population live (2022). https://www.worldometers.info/world-population/india-population/. Accessed 16 May 2022

AI Applied to COVID-19

Business Intelligence Platform for COVID-19 Monitoring: A Case Study

Ricardo Duarte[1] , João Lopes[1] , Tiago Guimarães[1(✉)] , Susana Ferreira[2], and Manuel Filipe Santos[1]

[1] ALGORITMI/LASI, University of Minho, Braga, Portugal
b12723@algoritmi.uminho.pt, {jlopes,tsg,mfs}@dsi.uminho.pt
[2] Centro Hospitalar Universitário do Porto, Porto, Portugal
sferreira@chporto.min-saude.pt

Abstract. With the emergence of the COVID-19 virus, the need to effectively and flexibly plan and manage the measures to be applied within a Healthcare institution has become imperative. New knowledge about the disease and legislative changes arose frequently and with high impacts on clinical practice and management.

The platform developed under this case study aggregates data from multiple sources within the Healthcare Institution and also from external entities, such as clinical analysis laboratories. Thus, it provides a set of dashboards that seeks to present in a simple and intuitive way, data analysis ranging from COVID tests and their results, bed occupancy, with an exceptional focus in occupancy in Intensive Care Units, to monitoring the positive movements of COVID patients in the *Centro Hospitalar e Universitário do Porto* (CHUP), in almost real time.

The development of this data collection, analysis and demonstration platform was created in response to a critical need for reliable information so that clinical and management decisions could be supported by solid foundations based on facts and current and reliable data.

Keywords: Business Intelligence · COVID-19 · Healthcare · Monitoring · ICU · Intensive Care

1 Introduction

The unprecedented global spread of SARS-COV-2, a virus that has become better known as COVID-19, has placed severe strains on hospital systems worldwide [1].

The unknown clinical features, together with the speed of viral spread, create a difficult situation in which healthcare professionals lack important diagnostic tools, such as accurate predictive models and data-based information on disease progression factors.

Intensive Care Units (ICU) became bigger and additional were created within each hospital so to respond to all needs.

J. M. Machado and H. Peixoto (Eds.): AISCOVID 2022, LNICST 485, pp. 41–50, 2023.
https://doi.org/10.1007/978-3-031-38204-8_4

Business Intelligence (BI) and Business Analytics (BA) technologies are increasingly being used to extract knowledge and turn it into useful information and analytical tools for healthcare professionals. These data-based tools are not only essential for healthcare providers in terms of risk prediction, but also play an essential role for policy makers in terms of resource allocation strategy, as they would be an asset for population distribution and vaccination planning. Such tools could help in identifying high-risk patients for first-line vaccines, in addition to priority groups and cancellations or rescheduling as they arise [2].

This document describes a BI system developed for the *Centro Hospitalar e Universitário do Porto* (CHUP), a Hospital in the north of Portugal, to allow health professionals the extraction of knowledge through data analysis, serving as support in the decision-making process. To obtain the solution, it was necessary to perform all the tasks associated with BA projects, to create dashboards with efficiency and quality indicators for COVID patients' management.

This work is divided into several sections, starting with a brief introduction. Section 2 presents a review of the literature on COVID-19 combined with BI. Sections 3 and 4 present the methodology used as well as the developed proposal, respectively. Finally, the final conclusions are presented.

2 Background

The COVID-19 outbreak started in November 2019 in Wuhan, China. In March 2020, the World Health Organization (WHO) declared a global pandemic. The COVID-19 virus is extremely infectious and has spread rapidly to every country in the world [3, 4]. Infection rates reached record levels and led to a high death rate. Countries have begun imposing lockdowns and curfews for the first time in decades. WHO has started campaigns to educate people about the importance of social distancing and wearing masks in public places. In parallel, scientists began to study the virus and develop accelerated vaccines. To date, there are six vaccines authorized by the World Health Organization, namely Pfizer-BioNTech, Moderna, Johnson & Johnson, Astrazeneca, Sputnik and Sinopharm [3].

For health organizations not to collapse and to be able to cope with this outbreak, it is necessary to improve the quality of health care provision. With a good understanding of the generated data, it directly reflects the success of the organization, because a good understanding of these, transforms them into useful information capable of improving its entire environment. When dealing with a huge amount of data, the task of understanding it without the use of technology becomes difficult. This is where BA tools come into play, as they offer a process capable of transforming raw data into useful information for the organization. In addition to providing an interactive and intuitive visualization of the most relevant information, facilitating its analysis and understanding. Consequently, it leads to an improvement in decision-making processes, executing decisions more thoughtful and efficient [5].

BI applications have been used to respond to existing needs in the industry. Governments and healthcare organizations should appreciate the use of these technologies to assist in tracking, monitoring, and controlling the pandemic, which includes the patient flow and vaccination process. The implementation of this system facilitates real-time communication, identifies any problems that may arise, and allows for better efficiency in the allocation of limited resources.

An intelligent system based on global knowledge must be incorporated to lead to a reliable vaccine delivery system. It follows the vaccine supply chain process from start to finish, that is, at all stages of the process. This includes the delivery process, and all the means used to follow up and monitor the entire process. In this way, assistance in scheduling vaccination appointments is improved, in addition to improved tracking and efficiency of vaccinations and vaccinated persons [3]. Control panels and charts are also essential and necessary for their implementation, as they are used to monitoring results and look for changes in processes. Applied to healthcare, control charts can be used to monitor outcomes such as patient status. Predicting disease transmission during an epidemic is a significant aspect of health management, as it helps to prevent and control disease transmission. Real-time climate data with the help of sensors, computing technologies and artificial intelligence were used to develop a big data-based surveillance system to monitor and control epidemics. The use of structured and unstructured hospital data, together with regional data, allows the construction of a strong forecasting model to help control the disease outbreak [6, 7].

3 Methodology

For the development of this solution, the Kimball methodology was used. The Ralph Kimball's methodological approach focuses on guiding the realization and development of projects with a Data Warehouse (DW), focusing on the needs and the data presented to users. Each implementation project must have a finite cycle with a specific beginning and end. A project management is carried out simultaneously, to follow the entire evolution of the solution, deadlines and duration [8]. Figure 1 shows all the phases of the Kimball's Methodology. The most important are described in the following chapter.

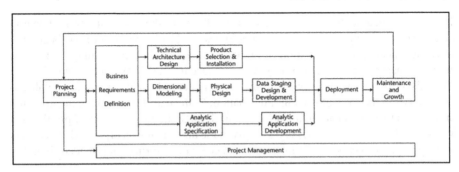

Fig. 1. Kimball's Methodology. Retrieved from [8].

4   Business Analytics Platform

Throughout this chapter, the phases of the Kimball methodology used to achieve the developed solution will be presented and described.

4.1 Project Planning

The project begins with the identification of development tasks to ensure its correct planning, meeting the defined deadlines. This product aims to develop a BI system to support health professionals at the CHUP, so that, through the visualisation of information and indicators, it allows better management of processes inherent to COVID-19 and all treatments to be provided to patients, accessing data with simplified and optimised visualisations to make decisions easier and more intuitive. Initially, the necessary tasks were identified and programmed, from the study of the available data to the design of solution, obtained by studying organisational requirements, understanding the data, data processing, ETL process and building the BI solution.

4.2 Business Requirements

The business requirements were defined, in order to identify the current needs that the CHUP has in the process of performance indicator management. Therefore, a study was carried out to determine what needs to be developed to meet the organisation's needs, being divided into functional and non-functional. These are:

1. Functional Requirements: Understand and implement performance indicators, such as the number of patients admitted, with clinical discharge, number of tests performed, flow of admissions over time, among others;
2. Non-functional Requirements: Intuitive solution, easy to interpret and access.

4.3 Technological Architecture

The technological architecture defined for the design of the final solution is shown in Fig. 1. The image illustrates all the technologies used and the process flow, beginning with the collection of information from different data sources, proceeding to the ETL process, where the data will be processed and loaded into a DW. When the data relates to the analysis tool, a visualization environment is created, which will be made available to the end user in the form of relevant information. Both areas developed are incorporated into the AIDABI application, a platform that, through the management of profiles and accesses, allows greater privacy and security of the information incorporated. Only users with appropriate access and permissions can access the information provided (Fig. 2).

4.4 Dimensional Modelling

Based on the existing data source, several relevant tables were selected to create a DW with the necessary dimensions and fact tables. The main objective of the fact tables is to manage the number of events regarding patients, collection results and hospitalisation

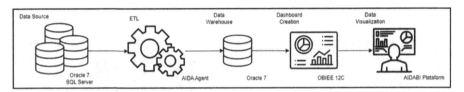

Fig. 2. Technological Architecture

flow. The dimensions contain all the important information to complement the existing information in the fact tables, highlighting patient demographics, tests performed, internal transfers, dates of occurrence and deaths. Before being loaded into the DW, all of them go through a data processing process, explained in the following sub-chapter.

4.5 Data ETL Design

When performing the analysis of the attributes that make up the different selected tables, some inconsistencies were identified, such as null values, excessive spacing between characters and spelling errors. The way to solve these problems is to replace the values by 0, eliminating the unnecessary spaces and replacing the errors by the correct nomenclature, respectively. All data processing operations are performed whenever new data is entered into the DW to maintain consistency in the type of data used in each of the dimensions and fact tables.

4.6 Analytical Application Development

The data presentation was carried out through dashboards in the Oracle BI tool. The solution is inserted and functioning at CHUP. It is a solution divided into two main components: Global data analysis and User interaction data analysis. In both, some additional columns and tables, metrics and filters were developed to control the visualizations and allow more robust and, consequently, more intuitive analysis. In the Global Data Analysis component, a series of dashboards were developed, each with its own specificities and contributions to the monitoring of COVID-19 within the institution. Each of the dashboards created are presented below, but only shown where data masking was reasonable:

1. **Synopsis** - Contains an overview of the evolution of the patient's status over time, by age group and condition. Additionally, it is possible to observe the status of hospitalizations and the evolution over time, stressing the number within ICU. The temporal evolution of accumulated cases per status is also shown, in addition to the number of collections made in the last 24 h.
2. **Occupancy and Hospitalization** - Displays the number of vacancies available for occupancy, the number of occupied beds and the current occupancy in the different hospital units. A special focus was given to ICU so to easily identify the number of occupied beds and vacancies within these units (Fig. 3).
3. **Recovered** - Contains a detailed list of patients who have been flagged as recovered, according to the criteria defined by the *Direção Geral de Saúde* (DGS).

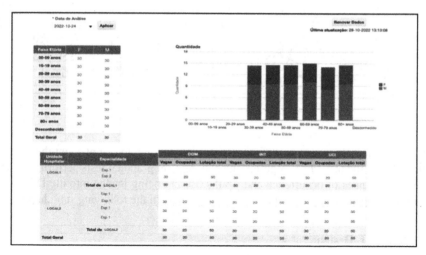

Fig. 3. Dashboard for data masked Occupancy and Hospitalization

4. **Deaths** - Displays a detailed listing of patients who tested positive for COVID-19, indicating the date on which their death was declared and the Length of stay for either regular internment, intensive care units or domicile.
5. **Clinical Analytics** - Contains the number of tests that each patient has performed. For each test performed it is possible to determine the module in which it was requested, the request date, the collection date and the result (which varies between Pending and the date in which it became available, a color being assigned to each of the states obtained) (Fig. 4).

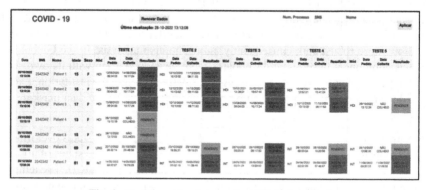

Fig. 4. Dashboard for data masked Clinical Analytics

6. **Patient Flow** - Shows the patient's evolution within the institution, i.e. from the moment they enter the CHUP until they leave. It is possible to see the specialties in which he/she has been, the place to which they belong, exams performed, admission and discharge date, as well as the episode registered (Fig. 5).

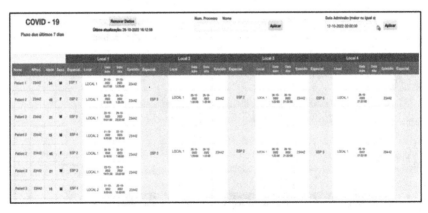

Fig. 5. Dashboard for data masked Patient Flow

7. **Geo** - Displays a geographical distribution by district of the number of positive cases, suspects and those awaiting the test result (Fig. 6).

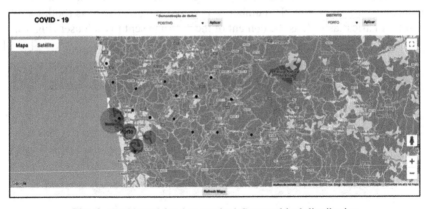

Fig. 6. Dashboard for data masked Geographical distribution

A series of dashboards were developed in the User interaction data analysis component, to maintain monitoring between the health institution and the patient about their status in relation to COVID-19. The dashboards developed are presented below:

1. **Webapp** - Some COVID positive patients whose symptoms were mild, were referred to confinement at home. In order to maintain a line of communication and constant monitoring of their symptoms, a web application was developed so that those patients could send daily updates of their health condition. Within this scope of data analysis, a dashboard was developed to administer and construe the data sent by the patients (Fig. 7).

2. **SMS monitoring panel** - CHUP sends a message to the patient about the result of the test performed within the institution and what to do if the test is positive. In the panel

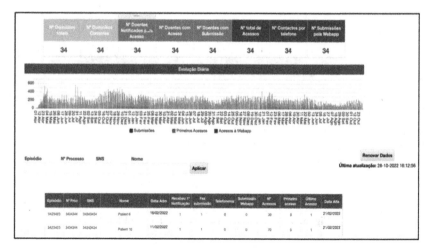

Fig. 7. Dashboard for data masked Webapp

developed for this monitoring, it is possible for the health institution to know the number of messages sent, the number of negative and positive tests (both for adults and Paediatrics) as well as the content of the message sent to each user (Fig. 8).

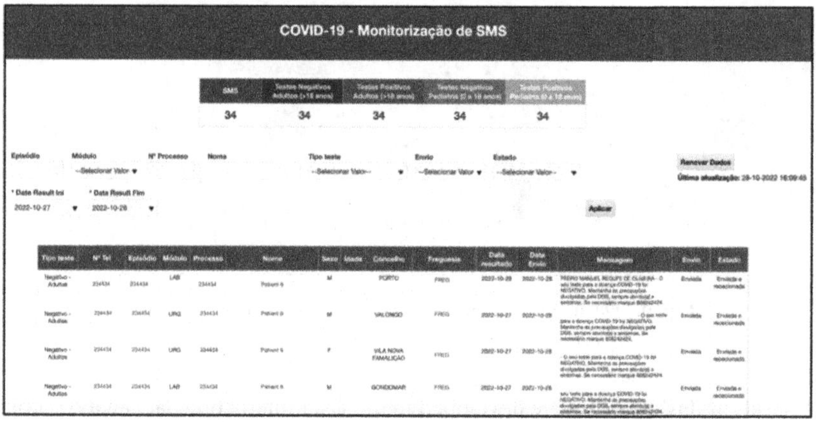

Fig. 8. Dashboard for data masked SMS monitoring

4.7 Implementation and Growth

The implementation of the final solution was carried out in different phases, initially ensuring the correct functioning of the technological structure implemented, followed by each of the dashboards prepared, allowing the validation of all information. Thus, in general, this process was divided into three different phases:

1. Phase 1: Testing of the prototype, to ensure proper functioning and integrity between the different functionalities;
2. Phase 2: Implementation of the final solution, with validation of the data and information presented;
3. Phase 3: Training for health professionals, encompassing the interaction with the platform, allowing them to learn and understand all the available information. It is necessary to guarantee the continuous growth of the developed solution with the appearance of new data and processes of the CHUP.

5   Conclusion and Future Work

The main goal of this project was to develop a BI system that would allow health professionals to extract knowledge through data analysis. The visualization interface presents a set of reports that have metrics capable of responding to the objectives and needs of the institution, with insights being provided in real time.

Areas like Intensive Care were a major focus within this conceptualization and implementation given the urgent need to monitor and optimize its usage and efficiency.

The pandemic forced a complete restructuring of several clinical processes, none of which could be done without access to important information for decision making. Thus, it is considered that the main contribution of this work comes from the logical capabilities of this platform, which is able to monitor, in real time, all the events inherent to COVID-19, with a functional solution implemented in the Health institution itself. Additionally, the research team was concerned with developing a solution capable of being optimized and adapted to other healthcare units, to improve the quality of care and user satisfaction.

As future work, new areas of information are being prepared, with the integration of new data sources, capable of including predictive analyses, to anticipate certain scenarios, such as the limit of admissions, resources, among others.

Acknowledgments. The work has been supported by FCT – Fundação para a Ciência e Tecnologia within the Projects Scope: DSAIPA/DS/0084/2018.

References

1. Izquierdo, J.L., Ancochea, J., Soriano, J.B.: Clinical characteristics and prognostic factors for intensive care unit admission of patients with COVID-19: retrospective study using machine learning and natural language processing. J. Med. Internet Res. **22**(10), 1–13 (2020). https://doi.org/10.2196/21801
2. Jimenez-Solem, E., et al.: Developing and validating COVID-19 adverse outcome risk prediction models from a bi-national European cohort of 5594 patients. Sci. Rep. **11**(1), 1–12 (2021). https://doi.org/10.1038/s41598-021-81844-x
3. Barakat, S., Al-Zagheer, H.: Business intelligence application in COVID-19 vaccine distribution. Ann. Rom. Soc. Cell Biol. **25**(6), 17973–17980 (2021). https://www.annalsofrscb.ro/index.php/journal/article/view/9161

4. Sen, S., Saha, S., Chatterjee, S., Mirjalili, S., Sarkar, R.: A bi-stage feature selection approach for COVID-19 prediction using chest CT images. Appl. Intell. **51**(12), 8985–9000 (2021). https://doi.org/10.1007/s10489-021-02292-8

5. Rocha, Á., Adeli, H., Reis, L.P., Costanzo, S., Orovic, I., Moreira, F. (eds.): WorldCIST 2020. AISC, vol. 1161. Springer, Cham (2020). https://doi.org/10.1007/978-3-030-45697-9

6. Ward, M.J., Marsolo, K.A., Froehle, C.M.: Applications of business analytics in healthcare. Bus. Horiz. **57**(5), 571–582 (2014). https://doi.org/10.1016/j.bushor.2014.06.003

7. Kamble, S.S., Gunasekaran, A., Goswami, M., Manda, J.: A systematic perspective on the applications of big data analytics in healthcare management. Int. J. Healthc. Manag. **12**(3), 226–240 (2019). https://doi.org/10.1080/20479700.2018.1531606

8. Kimball, R., Ross, M.: The data warehouse toolkit: the complete guide to dimensional modelling (2011)

First Clustering Analysis of COVID in Portugal

Ana Teresa Ferreira[1], José Vieira[2], Manuel Filipe Santos[1], and Filipe Portela[1,2(✉)]

[1] Algoritmi Research Centre, University of Minho, Guimarães, Portugal
cfp@dsi.uminho.pt
[2] IOTECH- Innovation on Technology, Trofa, Portugal

Abstract. There is an increasing need to understand the behavior of COVID-19, in this case, what type of medical preconditions can influence the recovery of the infected patient and what age groups are more affected. After the Directorate-General of Health of Portugal (DGS) made available the first records gathered from the infected, it became possible gather some conclusions. In this context, ioCOVID19 project arises, which wants to identify patterns and develop intelligent models able to support the clinical decision.

This article explores which typologies are associated with different outcomes to provide some insights regarding the consequences after the coronavirus infection. To understand which profiles, stand out, a clustering algorithm was used, 65 experiments were carried out, from which 192 clusters were obtained. From this study, the most relevant profiles are the following: the profile associated with death are patients with Diabetes – aged between 44 and 98 years old (19.74%); regrading hospitalized patients who died, the profile achieved was patients with Chronic Kidney Disease – aged between 52 and 102 years old (17.63%); for patients hospitalized in ICU who died the profile obtained was Cardiovascular Diseases – aged between 61 and 88 years old (26.23%); in regards to patients who died after being submitted to ventilatory support the correlated profile are patients with Cardiovascular Diseases – aged between 62 and 99 years old (32.17%). With the completion of this study it was possible to detect a set of profiles that are associated with different clinical conditions.

Keywords: COVID-19 · Clustering · Information Systems · Statistics · Public Health

1 Introduction

With the increase of severe acute respiratory syndrome coronavirus 2 (SARS-CoV-2) cases, it becomes necessary to understand what outcome can be gathered from the data collected by medical health professionals in the field. Portugal is one of the European Countries where Coronavirus has a significant impact, and the number of cases and deaths increase every day. To provide some inputs to the decision process, a research project was released – ioCOVID19 aims to develop an intelligent decision support platform that predicts the evolution of the disease in a specific patient. Providing support to clinicals

J. M. Machado and H. Peixoto (Eds.): AISCOVID 2022, LNICST 485, pp. 51–61, 2023.
https://doi.org/10.1007/978-3-031-38204-8_5

in the fight against COVID-19. Given that, this article was developed as an integral part of the research project depicted and its essentiality falls within the phase of Data Understanding and Preparation using data mining techniques.

The aim of the study is to understand the trends of the virus considering the preconditions and age of the infected. In this context, this work helps health professionals in the moments of crucial decision making – based on previous cases of infected patients who can provide some output regarding the outcome that may result. For this, clusters were created based on the characteristics of those affected. In this way, it's possible to understand in which group the infected patient may be inserted in and if these preconditions influence in any way progression of the disease (coronavirus). The data found in this article goes back to June of 2020 and refers only to the Portuguese population. At this moment according to Directorate-General of Health (DGS) of Portugal, the average age of deaths due to COVID-19 is 81.4 years old [1].

The article presents the following structure: first, to situate the reader in the theme and problem addressed, a short introduction to the subject is presented. Next, it's described with more detail what type of data mining technique are used during the study, and an analysis of the data is also provided. The main themes of the article are detailed in the Background section, as well as information related to previous studies developed about the same matter. Then, it is portrayed in more detail which materials and methods were used for the development of the project, such as which methodologies were adopted and what kind of data was utilized. Regarding the Case Study point, the first 3 phases of CRISP-DM are exposed in more detail based on the project's objective. Then, in the Modeling phase, all the relevant information used during the data clustering process is presented. In the section referring to the Results, all relevant results and information obtained during the creation of the clusters are exposed. Lastly, in the Discussion section, all results disclosed in the previous points are discussed and evaluated in detail in a critical way.

2   Background

This section presents the relevant topics of the article, shows the Portugal situation at the time, and mentions some related works.

2.1   COVID-19

COVID-19 is the official name given by the World Health Organization (WHO) to the disease caused by the new coronavirus SARS-CoV-2 (Severe acute respiratory syndrome coronavirus 2), which can cause a serious respiratory infection such as pneumonia. This virus was first identified in humans in the Chinese city of Wuhan, Hubei province, at the end of 2019 [2].

2.2   Portuguese Reality of COVID-19

According to official data, on June 30 of 2020, the scenario in which Portugal found itself was as follows: 42 171 confirmed cases, 27 505 recovered cases and 1 576 cases of death [3]. To better understand the effect of the pandemic in Portugal, the mortality rate of the coronavirus on June 30, 2020, and the deadliest diseases in the country. According to available data, for the year of 2019, the three most deadly diseases were the following [4]: Diseases of the circulatory system (represents 29,9% of deaths), Malignant tumors (25,5%) and Respiratory system diseases (10,9%). In contrast, on 30 June, the mortality rate due to COVID-19 was 3.74% [5].

2.3   Project ioCOVID19

The article in question is linked to the project under development - ioCOVID19 – Intelligent Decision Support Platform NORTE-01-02B7-FEDER-048344. It aims to create an essential platform for clinicians to combat COVID-19, and its main objective is to analyze the available data referring to those infected by coronavirus in Portugal and to predict the evolution of the disease of a given patient from a set of predictive models. Through the use of open data accessible online and made available by the SNS (Portuguese National Health Service) and DGS, it is possible to categorize the type of patients, assess the impact that each variable has on the course of the disease and predict the type of patient discharge. A Web/Mobile platform - ioCOVID19 - is also being developed, which aims to allow doctors/nurses to access a set of essential data for decision making.

2.4   Data Mining

Data Mining refers to the ability to extract useful and relevant information from a large dataset. In this study field, the main objective is to find non-evident relationship between data or patterns, in other words, it's the process of discovering knowledge from data [6] that can add some value to the dataset owner.

2.5   Clustering

Data clustering is a technique used in Data Mining, to provide statistical data analysis. Clustering is the classification of similar objects in different groups, that is the separation of data into clusters. The data inserted in each cluster, ideally, has some common trait [6]. In general, clustering is about identifying a finite set of categories or clusters do describe the data.

2.6   Similar Works

Since the study focuses on a relatively recent disease, no study like the one presented in this article was found. However, studies related with the clinical field have already been developed using the Clustering technique. That said, the studied found was the following:

- Identification of clusters of symptoms that can interfere in the quality of life of patients with advanced cancer, thus allowing greater control of them by clinicians, to reduce side effects in those patients [7].

- Identification of risk factors associated COVID-19 deaths in Portugal, in order to allow a more efficient health services strategic interventions with a significant impact on deaths by COVID-19 [8].

3   Materials and Methods

The portrayed data was provided by DGS and SNS. It refers to patients infected with COVID-19, collected by clinicals between 2nd March and 30th June of 2020.

3.1   Design Science Research

Since this is a research project and to understand if it's possible to characterize the clinical typology of patients infected with coronavirus (as well as the outcome of the disease), two methodologies were followed - Design Science Research (DSR), as a research methodology and Cross-Industry Standard Process for Data Mining (CRISP-DM) as practical method. DSR consists of 6 phases [9]:

1. Identifying the problem and motivation;
2. Defining objectives of the solution;
3. Design and development;
4. Demonstration;
5. Evaluation;
6. Communication.

To set DSR in action, it's necessary to use a practical methodology to help drive the project, so, CRISP-DM was chosen.

3.2   CRISP-DM

CRISP-DM was the second methodology used. This method provides a global perspective on the life cycle of a data mining project. This cycle, shown in Fig. 1 - Project Workflow - is divided into 6 sequential phases. There are dependencies between them; however, it does not have a rigid structure. The phases of the current CRISP-DM model for data mining projects are Business Understanding, Data Understanding, Data Preparation, Modelling, Evaluation and Deployment. The information depicted in this document was achieved after the completion of the third phase - Data Preparation [10]. Regarding that, there is a more detailed description of the phases involved.

To drive this project is essential to do a relation between the research methodology and the practical method.

3.3   DSR and CRISP-DM

Since both methodologies are used concurrently, it's possible to point out the relationship between the two. This article portrays the three first phases of both CRISP-DM and DSR. For example, phase 1 and 2 of the DSR are directly linked to the first activity of CRISP-DM, as portrayed in the table. The remaining correlations are also shown in Table 1 – Crossover of CRISP-DM and DSR methodologies [9].

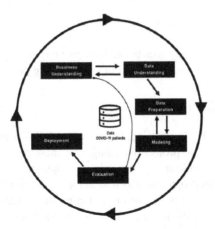

Fig. 1. Project Workflow

Table 1. Crossover of CRIPS-DM and DSR methodologies

Methodology	Activities	DSR Phases					
		1	2	3	4	5	6
CRISP-DM	Business Understanding	X	X				
	Data Understanding		X	X			
	Data Preparation			X			
	Modeling			X			
	Evaluation				X	X	
	Deployment				X	X	

3.4 Tools

To develop the project depicted, Python programming language was used. For such, to apply this language a set of libraries were applied to enable the preparation and the analysis of the data in question. The libraries employed were the following:

- Panda's library (allows the manipulation of data organized by columns);
- Matplotlib (provides different information visualization options);
- Scikit-learn or sklearn (is a machine learning software that provides various algorithms such as Classification, Regression and Clustering).

The Clustering algorithm used to support the study was K-Means Clustering. This algorithm seeks to divide all the observations under analysis into "k" clusters, with each observation belonging to the closest centroid. In this way, it's possible to survey observations that have some determining characteristic in each of the groups.

4 Case Study

The description of the case study goes through the methodology, presented in the CRISP-DM section, as it's possible to understand in the following points.

4.1 Business Understanding

The first phase, Business Understanding, focuses essentially on understanding the objectives and requirements of the project regarding a business perspective. From there, it's then possible to design a preliminary data mining project that can achieve the outlined objectives. Therefore, this project intends to develop a platform for clinicians to combat COVID-19, with the primary objective of predicting the evolution of the disease of a specific patient - evaluating the impact that each variable has on disease and predicting the type of outcome. For this study, the aim is to categorize the types of clinical patients in Portugal.

4.2 Data Understanding

At this stage, data analysis is carried out to search for possible quality problems and, consequently, obtain a better understanding of them. Since the data concerning COVID-19 was recorded by a wide range of health professionals, it was shown that it was inconsistent. The data provided has 38,545 records, which were collected between the 2nd of March and the 30th of June. To gather a better perception of the data, an annex - COVID-19 Data Analysis - was created where all the relevant information is exposed. Nevertheless, a global perception of the data is exposed in Table 2 – General Analysis:

Table 2. General Analysis

Study Groups	Number of records	% of records
Patients with Comorbidities	8326	21.60%
Admission	4327	11.23%
Deaths	1155	3.00%
Ventilatory Support	4327	11.23%
ICU Admission	253	0.66%
Recovered Patients	17 046	44.23%

4.3 Data Preparation

In this phase, all the changes applied are portrayed to build the final dataset, that is, the data that later is used to feed the modelling tools. The main tasks performed were cleaning data, selecting attributes, and building new attributes from existing data. Some of the main corrections/changes made were:

- The correction of fields that indicated pregnant men. This error was present in 3 records and represents 0.0078% of the data;
- Ignore records that precede the first confirmed official case in Portugal. This error was present in 23 records, which represented 0.060% of the data and were subsequently eliminated from the data;
- The creation of columns about other comorbidities through the column "If another, which one?" - such as the addition of the columns Cardiovascular Diseases, Obesity, Smoking, Tuberculosis, Rhinitis, Bronchitis, among others. This change affected 4970 columns, that is, 12.90% of the records.

5 Modeling

At this point, the entire process concerning the modelling and elaboration process of the clusters is exposed. To understand the best clustering algorithm to use, several have been studied and considered and several experiments were carried out to obtain the presented results and conclusions. That said, 33 experiments (3 Scenarios * 11 Targets * 1 Methods) were carried out and documented to better understand the preconditions or other factors such as gender, age, hospitalization, ICU service and the need for ventilatory support. Other experiments were also carried out to find the correlation between the various diseases under study, however, it wasn't possible to obtain relevant information on this point. In total 112 experiences were elaborated, which gives a total of 325 clusters. However, about half of these experiments refer to tests performed, to understand what kind of information and correlation it would be possible to extract from the data. Given that 33 experiments were then documented, as they were the ones that demonstrated to have relevant and usable information.

Therefore, the targets under consideration were as follows:

```
{
"Scenarios":{
        "S1":"All Comorbidities ",
        "S2":"Risk Comorbidities ",
        "S3":"Risk Comorbidities except Cardiovascular Diseases"
},
"Targets":{
        "TG1":"All infected people who died",
        "TG2":"All Hospitalized",
        "TG3":"All Hospitalized who died",
        "TG4":"Everyone who needed an Intensive Care Unit (ICU)",
        "TG5":"All who needed ICU and died",
        "TG6":"All infected who needed ventilatory support",
        "TG7":"All those infected who needed ventilatory support who died",
        "TG8":"All Recovered",
        "TG9":"All Hospitalized who recovered",
        "TG10":"All who needed ICU and recovered",
        "TG11":"All who needed ventilatory support and recovered"
},
"Methods":{
        "ALG1":"K - Means with Elbow Method"
}
}
```

Regarding all the mentioned targets, studies were carried out considering all the preconditions portrayed, all the preconditions considered at risk, all the risk preconditions (except for cardiovascular diseases), and risk preconditions with age or gender, however no relevant results were gathered by the last two, therefore, they were discarded. Comorbidities considered at risk are: Neoplasm, Diabetes, Human Immunodeficiency Viruses (HIV) and others Immunodeficiencies, Chronic neurological and/or Neuromuscular diseases (CNND), Asthma, Chronic Lung Disease, Hepatic pathology, Chronic Hematological Diseases, Chronic Kidney Disease, Chronic Neurological Disability, Obesity, Smoking and Cardiovascular Disease (since is considered the deadliest disease in Portugal.). However, as the designation of cardiovascular disease is very general (since it can represent more serious or less severe illnesses within the same branch), the study of risk comorbidities without this aspect was elaborated, to discover what other pre-conditions would also stand out.

To discover the most appropriate cluster number to be used for each target, the elbow method was used. This method analyses the percentage of variance explained as a function of the number in clusters. The first clusters add information but, after a certain point, the difference between the clusters decreases to the point of not adding relevant information. So, for the targets under study, with the help of the Elbow Method, it was found which number of clusters is the most appropriate and for the study in question, the number of clusters obtained varies from experience to experience. That said, the number of insured clusters varies between 2 and 4 clusters.

6   Results

In this section only the best results will be exposed. However, an annex - Clustering Results - with all collected clustering results will also be made available. Therefore, in Table 3 - "Best Clustering Results", the results of the attributes that demonstrate having some relevant information were exposed. For each target, the number and percentage of records for that target will be exposed, which scenario has obtained the best cluster, as well as, the affected ages, the highlighted disease and finally, from this sample, how many patients have the highlighted profile in the cluster.

Table 3. Best Clustering Results

Targets	N° and % of records	Scenarios	Affected Ages	Comorbidities	% of records per cluster
TG1	1155 (3.00%)	S1	[44–98]	Diabetes	19.74%
		S3	[52–100]	Chronic Kidney	13.25%
			[42–99]	Neoplasm	6.23%
TG3	72 (0.19%)	S1	[57–98]	CNND	10.33%
		S2	[52–100]	Chronic Kidney	17.63%
		S3	[44–95]	Neoplasm	13.64%
TG4	253 (0.66%)	S1	[18–92]	Cardiovascular Disease (C.D.)	30.04%
			[0–96]	Chronic Lung	11.46%
		S3	[0–96]	Chronic Kidney	13.83%
TG5	61 (1.28%)	S1	[61–88]	C.D	26.23%
		S3	[52–84]	Chronic Kidney	11.48%
TG6	493 (1.28%)	S1	[0–97]	C.D	59.63%
		S3	[51–94]	Chronic Lung	17.04%
TG7	115 (0.30%)	S1	[62–99]	C.D	32.17%
		S2	[56–91]	Chronic Lung	22.61%
		S3	[55–97]	Chronic Kidney	20.00%
TG8	17046 (44.22%)	S1	[25–99]	C.D	6.20%
		S3	[12–96]	Neoplasm	2.37%
TG9	1645 (4.27%)	S1	[12–100]	Diabetes	19.70%
		S3	[34–95]	Neoplasm	17.26%
TG10	81 (0.21%)	S3	[44–80]	Diabetes	35.80%
TG11	167 (0.43%)	S1	[44–97]	Diabetes	35.93%
		S3	[56–94]	Chronic Lung	16.17%

7   Discussion

As already portrayed, the aim of the study is to find different profiles of infected patient. From the results shown in the annex – Clustering Results – it's possible to identify Cardiovascular Diseases and Diabetes in all the targets studied. This is because, a significant percentage of the Portuguese population is affected by cardiovascular diseases, which naturally results in the highlight of this comorbidity in almost all targets studied. Because of this, it's not possible to associate patients who have this type of comorbidities (cardiovascular disease and diabetes), to a positive or negative outcome, since it presents itself in targets referring to patients who died, recovered, admitted, admitted to the ICU, etc. The highlighted comorbidities were as follows: Cardiovascular Disease, Diabetes, Chronic Kidney Disease, Neoplasm, Chronic Neurological and/or Neuromuscular, Chronic Lung Disease.

Regarding the Chronic Kidney Disease comorbidity, it's typically associated with patients over 52 years of age, and is present in the targets TG1 (13.25%), TG3 (17.63%), TG4 (13.83%), TG5 (11.48%), TG7 (20.00%), and all these targets are associated with patients who died, who needed hospitalization and/or died and needed ICU. As for the comorbidity Neoplasm, it is typically associated with patients older than 34 years, and is present in the following targets: TG1 (6.23%), TG3 (13.64%), TG8 (2.37%) and TG9 (17.26%), that is, it's related with patients who required hospitalization, but does not have a specific outcome, since it is present in patients who have died and who have recovered. About Chronic Neurological and/or Neuromuscular Disease, it's present in patients between 57 and 98 years old, who required hospitalization and died, that is, associated with TG3 (10.33%). Finally, for Chronic Lung Disease, it's typically in patients over 50, who needed ICU, ventilatory support, being present both in patients who required ventilatory support who recovered or died, in other words correlated with the targets TG4 (11.46%), TG6 (17.04%), TG7 (22.61%), TG11 (16.17%).

8   Conclusion

The study depicted represents only a part of the ioCOVID19 project in development, and any updates to the results set out in this article can be found on the project's website. Important to remember that the results obtained represent only a small sample of patients infected by COVID-19 in Portugal, since it is an analysis of the first data provided.

Hereupon, it was possible to outline different types of patients with the data provided, that is, the aim of the project was achieved. So, from the clustering investigation carried out and evaluation of the results obtained it was assessed which comorbidities were associated with each target. That said, the main conclusions, in summary form, after the analysis of the data by the clustering technique were that the Chronic Kidney Disease, is mostly associated with targets that resulted in the patient's death, Neoplasia is associated with patients who needed hospitalization and Chronic Lung Disease is mostly associated with patients who have ICU or ventilatory support. However, it was not possible to outline a profile for patients with Diabetes and Cardiovascular diseases, since they are present in all targets studied. In the exposed article, only the most relevant results were portrayed, the interested reader should consult the official page of the project for more information, https://iocovid19.research.iotech.pt/.

Acknowledgements. This work has been developed under the scope of the project NORTE-01-02B7-FEDER-048344, supported by the Northern Portugal Regional Operational Programme (NORTE 2020), under the Portugal 2020 Partnership Agreement, through the European Regional Development Fund (FEDER). This work has also been supported by FCT – Fundação para a Ciência e Tecnologia within the R&D Units Project Scope: UIDB/00319/2020.

References

1. DGS COVID-19 homepage. https://covid19.min-saude.pt/media-de-idades-dos-obitos-por-covid-19-e-81-4-anos/. Accessed 14 May 2021
2. COVID-19 | SNS24 [Internet]. SNS24. 2020 [cited 27 October 2020]. https://www.sns24.gov.pt/tema/doencas-infecciosas/covid-19/
3. Relatório de Situação. In: COVID-19. https://covid19.min-saude.pt/relatorio-de-situacao/. Accessed 14 May 2021
4. Óbitos por algumas causas de morte (%). In: Pordata.pt. https://www.pordata.pt/Portugal/%C3%93bitos+por+algumas+causas+de+morte+(percentagem)-758. Accessed 14 May 2021
5. Sete gráficos com a evolução da covid-19. Doentes internados em máximos de dois meses. In: Jornaldenegocios.pt. https://www.jornaldenegocios.pt/economia/coronavirus/detalhe/sete-graficos-com-a-evolucao-da-covid-19-em-portugal-taxas-de-crescimento-com-tendencia-de-queda. Accessed 14 May 2021
6. Bharati, M., Ramageri, M.: Data mining techniques and applications (2010)
7. Walsh, D., Rybicki, L.: Symptom clustering in advanced cancer. Support Care Cancer **14**, 831–836 (2006)
8. Nogueira, P.J., et al.: The role of health preconditions on COVID-19 deaths in portugal: evidence from surveillance data of the first 20293 infection cases. J. Clin. Med. **9**, 2368 (2020)
9. Fernandes, G.: Pervasive Data Science Applied to the Services Society. Master's Thesis, University of Minho, Guimarães, Portugal (2019)
10. Wirth, R., Hipp, J.: CRISP-DM: towards a standard process model for data mining. In Proceedings of the 4th International Conference on the Practical Applications of Knowledge Discovery and Data Mining, Manchester, UK, 1–13 April 2000

Multichannel Services for Patient Home-Based Care During COVID-19

Ailton Moreira[1]([✉])[iD], Maria Salazar[2][iD], Cesar Quintas[2][iD],
and Manuel Filipe Santos[1][iD]

[1] ALGORITMI Research Centre/LASI, University of Minho, Guimarães, Portugal
ailton.moreira@algoritmi.uminho.pt, mfs@dsi.uminho.pt
[2] Centro Hospitalar Universitário do Porto, Porto, Portugal
{msalazar,cesar.quintas}@chuporto.min-saude.pt

Abstract. At the beginning of 2020, the Worldwide Health Organization (WHO) declared a pandemic caused by the COVID-19 virus. In this
sense, this article describes an experiment carried out in a Portuguese
health institution during the COVID-19 pandemic between March and
July 2020. The number of cases of infection increased exponentially
and health facilities were forced to adapt to the circumstances. Due to
the health facility limited resources they had to be innovative. A new
modality of care service was introduced in which patients were admitted
to home-based care to receive medical follow-up. The modality introduced focuses mainly on multichannel interaction between patients and
health professionals. Two channels of interaction were made available to
patients in home-based care to interact with health professionals. Also,
a back-office platform was designed to support health professionals in
the management of patients diagnosed with the disease and all the processes related to patient remote follow-up and their decision-making. The
results of the experiments were very positive with the modality implemented both for patients and care facilities and their health professionals.
The patients were able to receive medical follow-up at their houses without any major complications and they were included in their treatment
process. The care facility was able to better manage and reallocate their
resource according to their need. This modality proved to be a win-win
situation for all the parties involved.

Keywords: Multichannel Services · Remote Patient Follow-up ·
COVID-19 · Healthcare Services

1 Introduction

The COVID-19 pandemic has increasingly reinforced the need for healthcare
institutions to find better ways to deal with patients in home-based care [25].
Currently, patients who do not need continuous and particular medical care,

Supported by organization CHUP.

ICST Institute for Computer Sciences, Social Informatics and Telecommunications Engineering 2023
Published by Springer Nature Switzerland AG 2023. All Rights Reserved
J. M. Machado and H. Peixoto (Eds.): AISCOVID 2022, LNICST 485, pp. 62–78, 2023.
https://doi.org/10.1007/978-3-031-38204-8_6

are admitted to home-based care [7]. Before the pandemic, mainly patient with diabetes was admitted to home-based care when they didn't require particular and in-person medical care. With the pandemic, this situation had a significant change [9,11], as patients that didn't require in-person treatment are admitted to home-based care. This practice has numerous advantages for both the healthcare institution and their health professional and the patients [10].

The present article focuses on a modality of multichannel interaction for remote patient monitoring implemented during COVID-19 at Centro Hospitalar Universitário do Porto (CHUP) [14]. Due to the high number of infected patients with SARS-COV-2 and with the limited resources healthcare facilities had, they had to be innovative and find new ways to provide care services to all the patients who had tested positive for COVID-19. One of the solutions found was the possibility of admitting to home-based care the patients who didn't have any symptoms caused by COVID-19. With this modality, patients could stay at home and still be followed by health professionals. In this sense, when patients tested positive for COVID-19 and hadn't any symptoms they were admitted to home-based care. They were given some instructions on how that modality works and instructions about the channels that they could use to interact with health professionals. The modality implemented had two channels of interaction (telephone contact and CHUP Monit) available to patients in home-based care [15]. With these two channels, patients could interact with health professionals and they could receive medical follow-up without the need to be in-person at health facilities. Also, at the health facilities, health professionals had a back-office platform to monitor the patient in home-based care and evaluate their clinical data.

To validate the applied modality, a research question was outlined for this article: **Was the use of multichannel services able to meet the needs of the patients while they were under medical surveillance?**

Thus, this article seeks to investigate and comprehend whether the patient's needs were met while they were under medical surveillance in home-based care during the COVID-19 pandemic.

This article is structured in seven sections. First, an introduction to the topic is made. Secondly, a background is presented. In the third section, the materials and methods used are described. Section four presents the implementation process of the multichannel services, as well as the applications developed. In five, the results are presented. Lastly, discussion and conclusions are drawn.

2   Background

Marketing and e-commerce organizations have been implementing different solutions for multichannel interaction with their customers and potential new customers [1,23]. This fact motivates us to design, propose, and implement a multichannel solution in healthcare services that enable patient interaction with health professionals across multiple channels.

Multichannel interaction in healthcare services is just getting started, with health institutions increasingly focusing on patients and the care services they provide [17]. In this regard, how health institutions interact and communicate with their patients is critical for a positive user experience for both patients and the health professionals who provide these care services. Multichannel interaction solutions have played an important role in ensuring that patients receive the service they expected and that health professionals can provide these services in the best working conditions in this process of communication and interaction between the two parties for the provision of care services [13,16]. Several studies and pilot projects have been implemented in recent years with new concepts and models tailored to the needs of each institution [3,7,10,11]. This article is based in multichannel conceptual model proposed for healthcare services by Ailton et al. (2020) [15,17].

Multichannel interaction services in a healthcare environment can bring many benefits for patients and health institution, by allowing the patient to use his/her preferred channel to communicate with the health institution. Patients value more health entity that interacts with them through their favourite channels. It also provides them with custom and personalized services according to their needs. Some key benefits of multichannel interaction in healthcare services were identified [4,24]:

- Increase patients satisfaction and patients relationship with healthcare entity;
- Target specific patients through their preferred channel with personalized services;
- Monitor and follow-up patients through multiple channels;
- Increase healthcare business.

Multichannel services in healthcare are an asset to patients as well as the health institution, but this paradigm shows some challenges that need to be overcome to successfully implement and tap the full potential of this paradigm. The challenges of delivering services across multiple channels in healthcare are diverse, varying from patient-related challenges, IT infrastructure and data protection and security, and privacy as well as healthcare-related challenges to communicate with patients in a multichannel interaction environment, such as [14,18]:

- Ensuring the continuous flow of communication between multiple channels;
- Data protection and privacy issues;
- Heterogeneous IT integration across multiple channels;
- Data integration across different channels.

2.1 Agency for Integration, Diffusion and Archive of Medical Information (AIDA)

AIDA is an interoperability platform specifically designed to solve the problem of integrating information from multiple systems based on multi-agent technologies that make an Health Information System (HIS) interoperable [2]. AIDA's platform consists of several modules with different functionalities and characteristics, all based on the interoperability of services and devices [6]. Since it was developed by a research group at the University of Minho, AIDA is already the main tool that guarantees interoperability in several Portuguese health organizations.

AIDA platform had a fundamental role in the multichannel model proposed and implemented during the first wave of COVID-19 at CHUP. As an interoperability platform, it ensures all communication among different HIS and data sharing across these systems. Also, it ensures that the data that the patients had registered is available and is presented to a health professional timely and organized to simplify their decision-making process.

3   Materials

The data used in this article were collected from the *Centro Hospitalar Universitário do Porto* (CHUP), which was a pilot experience with the implementation of a multichannel interaction solution in healthcare services during the first wave of the pandemic. These data pertain to patients who tested positive for COVID-19 but did not show any symptoms (asymptomatic patients) and were admitted for home-based care due to resource and health professional limitations at CHUP. The focus of this article will be solely on patients admitted for home-based care and their interactions with health professionals during the period of medical surveillance.

Table 1. COVID-19 numbers at CHUP

Indicators	Total
Patients with COVID 19 at CHUP	1794
Patients in Home-based Care	862
Patient Interactions	12605
CHUP Monit	11612
Telephone Contact	993

The COVID-19 data collected between March and July 2020 is displayed in Table 1. A total of 1794 COVID-19 patients were admitted to the hospital during that time. 862 patients (48%) didn't exhibit several symptoms, thus they didn't require in-person medical care. These patients were ultimately admitted to home-based care to avoid overloading the care facility resources. They had two ways to communicate with the health professionals that were monitoring their health conditions at home-based care. In total, they had 12612 interactions while receiving home-based care, of which 11612 (92,18%) interactions occurred via CHUP Monit (a web application made specifically for these patients to log their SARS-COV2-related symptoms), and 993 (7,88%) interactions occurred via a telephone contact that was made available to these patients to engage in direct communication with the accompanying health professional.

To perform the analysis of the data obtained a quantitative method of analysis was chosen as the data gathered were presented in numerical format. The quantitative method fits better as it allows to apply of some statistical analysis to the data collected.

4   Multichannel Services Implemented During COVID-19

First, it is presented a simplified version of the COVID-19 workflow implemented at CHUP before discussing the multichannel model implemented.

4.1   COVID-19 Workflow

Patients who did not have severe COVID-19 symptoms were admitted for home-based care for the hospital to better manage its resources [22]. Figure 1 depicts, in a simplified form, the hospital workflow in the context of COVID-19 emergencies. The focus of this article will be on the interaction channels that patients use to communicate with health professionals. Patients admitted to home-based care were given two channels to communicate with health professionals: CHUP Monit and a telephone contact that allowed patients to intercommunicate directly with the health professionals who were monitoring them.

- **CHUP Monit** - web application designed specifically for patients admitted for home-based care to interact with health professionals and track the evolution of symptoms caused by the COVID-19 virus while they were under medical surveillance.
- **Telephone Contact** - patients admitted to home-based care were given a phone number to contact health professionals directly as an alternative channel of interaction with health professionals while they were under medical supervision.

These two channels enabled health professionals to follow-up the patients as the symptoms caused by the COVID-19 virus evolved. The workflow starts with the initial contact with CHUP (telephone referral or emergency) and continues with attendance at the COVID-19 service, triage, and referral to hospitalization or home-based care, in case of patient had low level of severity or lack of symptoms.

Patients admitted for home-based care continued to receive medical monitoring and follow-up. When these patients do not show any further symptoms for a specified period or test negative for the SARS-CoV-2 virus or fulfilled the health-care regulatory restrictions, they had a medical discharge. As stated before, this paper will focus on the last part of the workflow designed for the channels used by patients during the period that they were under medical surveillance.

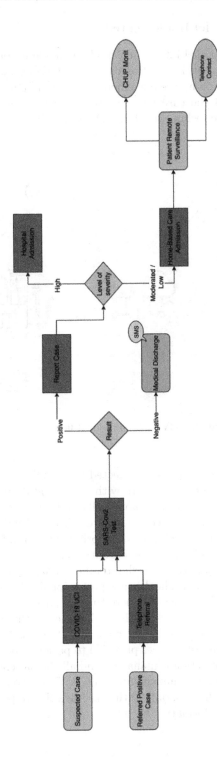

Fig. 1. COVID-19 simplified flow

4.2 Multichannel Model Implemented

The implemented multichannel interaction model is made up of three tiers: the patient tier with the respective interaction channels, the coordination tier, which handles all of the integration and management of the data made available in the interaction channels, and the care provider tier, which accommodates health professionals and all of the technological infrastructure that is part of the model presented [15,17] (Fig. 2).

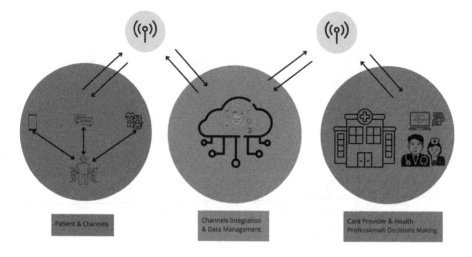

Fig. 2. COVID-19 simplified flow

- **Patient Tier** - this tier has patients infected with COVID-19 and the channels available to them to communicate with the hospital and health professionals. The available channels are phone calls, web app, and SMS. Patients use these available channels to communicate with healthcare professionals when they need them, to get help, or to get other types of information about their health condition, and to make a self-surveillance.
- **Coordination Tier** - this tier, coordinate and manage all the information made available to patients and healthcare professionals. This tier is the core of the solution proposed because it is here that all patient data management is carried out, as well as in ensuring, the persistence of these data and their safety in different channels used by patients. This tier was crucial for all the interaction and continuity of services provided to patients, because is through this tier that all the interaction is managed, and all the patient health records are available in this tier. It is implemented in CHUP due to data privacy and data protection issues. Besides, only authorized healthcare professionals have access to this tier and information on it.

– **Care Provider Tier** - this tier is the CHUP where the solution is implemented and all healthcare professionals who use the solution to follow-up and monitor patients with COVID-19 from nurses, doctors, and laboratory technicians, among others. Also, this tier is where all the technological infrastructure that supported the proposed solution is implemented. All the information processed, the databases, as well as the defined logical and business rules, are kept in this tier at CHUP to ensure and guarantee the privacy and protection of the patient's clinical data.

The CHUP Monit and the telephone contact used by patients are represented on the patient tier. To manage, integrate and present all the patient clinical data, a web app was designed to meet these needs. That web app was supported by many HIS and the AIDA platform. AIDA had an important role here as it used its intelligent agents to guarantee the interoperability of data to be presented to health professionals and patients [2, 19]. The AIDA platform was represented on the coordination tier. All the systems and applications used to implement the multichannel solution during the experiment carried out were implemented at the care provider tier. Physically both the coordination tier and care provider tier are located at the same facility. Also, the care provider tier is where is located all the health professionals that interact with the patient through multiple channels of interaction.

4.3   CHUP Monit

Following a diagnosis of COVID-19 virus infection, the treating physician evaluates the patient's status to determine if he/she may receive treatment at home for moderate and low symptoms or whether he/she has to be hospitalized for severe symptoms. Doctor follow-up is required daily for patients receiving home-based care. To speed up this procedure, a new web app was designed, allowing patients to communicate self-monitoring data.

Thus, the CHUP Monit was projected. It was a responsive web app, conceived to be used on mobile devices by patients in home-based care. It was a simple application but with an important role in patient self-monitoring and follow-up. It had fill two main requirements which are to allow patients to register their symptoms caused by COVID-19, and allow them to have access to the history of all the data of self-monitoring registered, with high level of security and data privacy. Figure 3 presents the CHUP Monit.

To proceed with the self-monitoring, the patients had to fill out a form with the evolution of their health status for medical follow-up during the home-based care internment. The following image demonstrates the records made by the patient about their health status with symbology that aid the data interpretation by health professionals.

Access to the patients was granted via the mobile phone number associated with the patient, who received a code via SMS for authentication. Besides, clear procedures were implemented to promote the efficient use of the web app. Whenever a new patient was admitted to home-based care, it was verbally informed

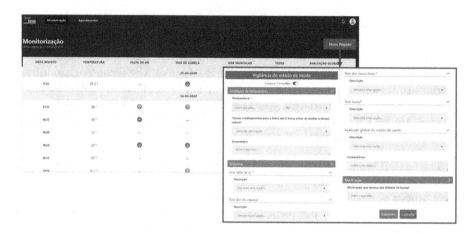

Fig. 3. CHUP Monit platform

to them and handed an informed leaflet about the two channels they can use to communicate with health professionals.

The patients who have used the web app to communicate with doctors recovered from the previous clinical condition in a shorter time and sent at least one update of the symptoms per day. They have been contacted whenever the clinical condition required and received orientations to act (e.g. medications, procedures).

The web app CHUP Monit allowed alternative communication channels by developing and making use of an online platform to interact asynchronously with patients and collect symptom data. Besides, the forms used were modeled according to open standards specifications, such as openEHR, FHIRE/HL7, and SNOMED-CT for data coding and modeling, and for interoperation with internal and external information systems [12, 14, 20, 21].

4.4   Telephone Contact

Patients admitted to home-based care had an additional method of communicating with health professionals in addition to the CHUP Monit. This channel was a telephone contact to have direct contact with health professionals. Through this, channel patients could chat with health professionals and relate to them their health condition and the symptoms that they were having. This was an asynchronous channel through which patients could have physitians' feedback at the same time.

4.5   Aida Contingency

As a back-office platform, Aida Contingency was designed to support health professionals' activities during the COVID-19 pandemic. This module is a web application with the purpose to manage COVID-19 workflow in different contexts and fields at CHUP. It had to be adapted due to the new coronavirus to accompany and monitor patients with COVID-19 from the moment they make the first contact with the hospital with possible symptoms of the virus until they had a medical discharge.

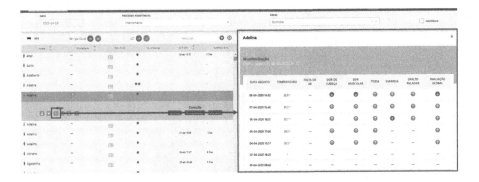

Fig. 4. AIDA Contingency platform

In a nutshell, AIDA Contingency enables health professionals to continuously monitor and follow-up infected patients through multiple channels of interaction remotely. Figure 4 shows the visualization of the monitoring report performed by a patient. Thus, the health professional can monitor the evolution of the patient's health condition and get in touch with him/her, if necessary. Aida Contingency was a complementary platform designed for health professionals to follow-up patients in home-based care. Through this platform, health professionals had access to all the patient records registered through CHUP Monit. The data is presented to health professionals very organized in order to make easier the health professional decision-making process.

5 Results

This section presents the main findings gathered from the data collected and a brief analysis of these data.

The chart presented in Fig. 5 shows that patients preferred to use the digital channel instead of the manual channel to interact with health professionals. The CHUP Monit was by far the preferred communication channel for patients to interact with healthcare professionals, given its portability and ease of use, combined with the low waiting time to interact with health professionals.

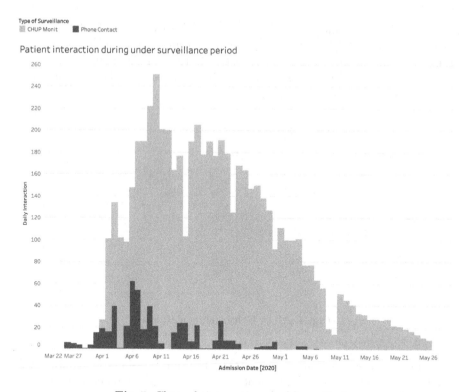

Fig. 5. Channels interaction used by patients

The chart presented in Fig. 6 contains information about channel utilization by patient age group. Based on this chart, it's possible to relate patients' channel utilization by each age group. Patients in the age group between 19 and 75 years old were the ones which had more interaction with health professionals as the difference between the channels used was very high.

The CHUP Monit was the patient's preferred channel of communication, as seen in the preceding Fig. 5. Based on Fig. 6, it is feasible to conclude that CHUP Monit (web app) was the channel that patients used the most to interact with health professionals across all age groups. Health practitioners didn't have to exert much effort to communicate with patients because telephone contact represents a relatively tiny share of interactions in each age group. Only when patients weren't utilizing the CHUP Monit or when the patient needed a medical discharge did they need to communicate with them over the telephone contact. The chart also highlights how crucial it is for patients to have access to a digital channel for communicating with medical practitioners. The use of digital channels reduces the health professionals' workload to follow-up with the patients at home-based care. Overall, despite the large age difference between patients, the CHUP Monit was the preferred interaction channel for patients to interact with health professionals, and it was well accepted by patients in general.

Multichannel interaction by group age

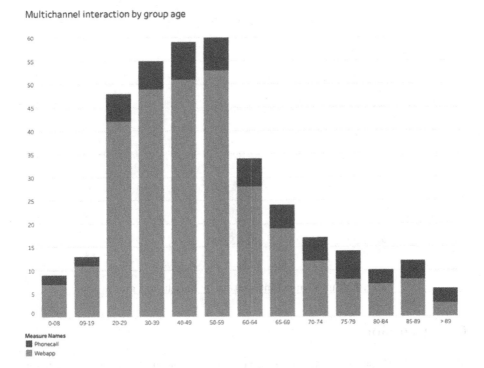

Fig. 6. Multichannel interaction by patient age group

Figure 7 illustrates the crossing made between channel utilization for a more in-depth analysis of the data gathered. The percentage of patients who only used the CHUP Monit to interact with health professionals (approximately 71,11%), the percentage of patients who only used telephone contact to interact with health professionals (approximately 4,47%), and the percentage of patients who used both channels of interaction (approximately 24,43%) were identified on Fig. 7.

An intriguing finding was that the use of both channels (CHUP Monit and telephone contact) was not proportional, but rather complementary, particularly in terms of decision-making by health professionals. When health professionals interacted with patients over the telephone contact, they maintained synchronous communication, which was more effective and efficient in providing information about the evolution of patients' symptoms and making decisions regarding medical discharge, or not, depending on the evolution of the symptoms.

The next section contains a brief overview of the findings derived from the data obtained, as well as the answer to the research question previously outlined for this article.

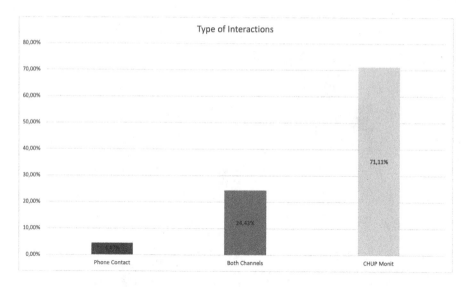

Fig. 7. Multichannel interaction by patient age group

6   Discussion

The COVID-19 pandemic has demonstrated that the digitization of health services is a trend that will continue, and more healthcare institutions are following suit by broadening the scope of care services they provide to their patients through different channels of interaction.

The objective of this study was to assess if patients undergoing home-based care follow-up during the COVID-19 pandemic had their requirements fulfilled. To do this, the gathered data was analyzed and some charts were prepared.

Although the idea of telemedicine or remote medical treatment is not new, it has gained popularity with the pandemic and more health institutions are adopting it as a strategy to follow. There are many models of telemedicine service for adoption today, each tailored to the requirements of healthcare institutions [8,11].

In the case of the multichannel interaction model proposed in CHUP during the pandemic, together with the analysis of the data collected as well as the feedback from patients and health professionals, it was a very positive experience for all parties involved and there were significant gains with this implementation.

The use of two interaction channels also made it possible for patients to always be in contact with health professionals in the moments they needed. Through CHUP Monit, patients could report the symptoms they were experiencing. In case the patients had any doubts they had a telephone contact to call and clarify their doubts with health professionals. Due to the availability of these channels and the simplicity of using them together with the feedback from the patients and the analysis of the data, some conclusions were outlined. With the availability and use of the two channels of interaction was possible to fulfill the patient's needs during the period they were under medical surveillance.

The use of digital channels (CHUP Monit) had a huge impact, and according to the charts presented in Fig. 5, 6, and 7, it is plausive to state that CHUP was the channel that had more utilization. This is because it had some key advantages when compared with the other channel (telephone contact) such as ease of use, no waiting time to make self-monitoring, and patients could make their self-monitoring at any time without any difficulties. The automation process implemented with the multichannel interaction model proposed on the self-monitoring process through CHUP Monit had a huge impact on the health professional workload on patient monitoring. With the digital channel, the patient's clinical data was presented to the health professional and they only had to analyze these data and make their decision. With the other channel (telephone contact) health professionals have to make manual contact with the patients to ask them about the symptoms that they were feeling at that moment. Without the CHUP Monit, this could require a huge effort of resource allocation by health institutions to follow-up with all the patients in home-based care.

Despite the CHUP Monit having more adherence and use it was less effective when compared with other channels. It was less effective because the patients didn't have direct contact with the health professional while with another channel (telephone contact) the patients had direct contact with the health professional and they could ask their questions and doubts and have their answers at that moment. Contrary to CHUP Monit this wasn't the case.

Besides many studies carried out present similar conclusions regarding the use of different channels of interaction to communicate with a health professional [3,5,10,11].

7   Conclusions

The realization of this article as well as the conclusions drawn from the data analysis came to reinforce even more that the multichannel service is here to stay in healthcare and that it can bring significant gains to the health institution.

There was a good acceptance by health professionals as it significantly reduced the level of effort required to carry out daily monitoring and manage patients during home-based care, by providing meaningful data to support quality clinical decision-making. On the other hand, from a total of 12605 interactions, only 993 (7.88%) were carried out by telephone contact. This means that approximately 92,12% of the time that professionals would have been devoted to contacting patients by telephone contact was freed up for other tasks.

There was a significant adherence of patients to the use of CHUP Monit to interact with health professionals since they felt that they were being part of the process and that they maintained direct contact with health professionals through the two interaction channels made available to them. Each one of the 862 patients in home-based care followed received an indication regarding how to use the CHUP Monit and to promote the use of the digital channel. Of these, 688 patients adhered to the CHUP Monit and, of these, 617 effectively reported their symptoms through the CHUP Monit (90%), which corresponds to a significant adherence.

In general, it was noted that there was a great gain in terms of interaction between the different stakeholders. The continuous interaction among the different stakeholders came to further strengthen the relationship between them and the consequent trust in the services that health professionals were providing to patients in home-based care [8,25].

The multichannel modality implemented during the first wave of COVID-19 at CHUP showed the potential that multichannel interaction has on healthcare services. Also, it showed some key contributions that these benefits have such as better resource allocation, reduced health professional workload, timely availability of patient clinical data, continuous communication between patients and health professionals, patient involvement during the treatment process, and many more. The patients were very pleased with the CHUP Monit as it allowed them to receive medical monitoring at their homes, and made them a part of all the medical care surveillance. Overall, they were very satisfied was the modality implemented and their feedback was positive with the use of both channels available to them, mainly the CHUP Monit due to the capabilities that it had.

In this article, an aspect that must be considered by health institutions whenever they deliver care services in the different channels of interaction was addressed, which is to ensure that they can meet the needs of their patients in the services that are provided to them with the use of information and communication technologies.

As mentioned previously the multichannel interaction in healthcare is in its early stage of adoption. The experiments carried out with the proposed model for multichannel interaction were successful, but it still has more space to be improved. In future work, the proposed model could be improved and more studies could be performed to address other key characteristics of multichannel interaction in healthcare services.

Acknowledgments. This work has been supported by "FCT-Fundação para a Ciência e Tecnologia" within the R&D Units Project Scope: UIDB/00319/2020. Alton Moreira has been supported by grant 2022.10342.BD.

References

1. Brown, J.R., Dant, R.P.: The role of e-commerce in multi-channel marketing strategy. In: Martínez-López, F.J. (ed.) Handbook of Strategic e-Business Management. PI, pp. 467–487. Springer, Heidelberg (2014). https://doi.org/10.1007/978-3-642-39747-9_20
2. Cardoso, L., Marins, F., Portela, F., Santos, M., Abelha, A., Machado, J.: The next generation of interoperability agents in healthcare. Int. J. Environ. Res. Public Health **11**, 5349–5371 (2014). https://doi.org/10.3390/ijerph110505349
3. Chunara, R., et al.: Telemedicine and healthcare disparities: a cohort study in a large healthcare system in New York city during COVID-19. J. Am. Med. Inform.

Assoc. **28**, 33–41 (2021). https://doi.org/10.1093/JAMIA/OCAA217. https://academic.oup.com/jamia/article/28/1/33/5899729

4. Coelho, F.J., Easingwood, C.: Multiple channel systems in services: pros, cons and issues. Serv. Ind. J. **24**(5), 1–29 (2004). https://doi.org/10.1080/0264206042000276810. https://www.tandfonline.com/action/journalInformation?journalCode=fsij20

5. Delana, K., Deo, S., Ramdas, K., Subburaman, G.B.B., Ravilla, T.: Multichannel delivery in healthcare: the impact of telemedicine centers in Southern India. Manag. Sci. (2022). https://doi.org/10.1287/mnsc.2022.4488

6. Duarte, J., et al.: Data quality evaluation of electronic health records in the hospital admission process. In: International Conference on Computer and Information Science (ACIS), pp. 201–206 (2010). https://doi.org/10.1109/ICIS.2010.97

7. Flumignan, C.D.Q., da Rocha, A.P., Pinto, A.C.P.N., Milby, K.M.M., Batista, M.R., Atallah, A.N., Saconato, H.: What do cochrane systematic reviews say about telemedicine for healthcare? Sao Paulo Med. J. **137**, 184–192 (2019). https://doi.org/10.1590/1516-3180.0177240419

8. Funderskov, K.F., Danbjørg, D.B., Jess, M., Munk, L., Zwisler, A.D.O., Dieperink, K.B.: Telemedicine in specialised palliative care: healthcare professionals' and their perspectives on video consultations-a qualitative study. J. Clin. Nurs. **28**, 3966–3976 (2019). https://doi.org/10.1111/JOCN.15004

9. Hak, F., Abelha, A., Santos, M.: Open science in pandemic times: a literature review. Procedia Comput. Sci. **177**, 552–555 (2020)

10. Haleem, A., Javaid, M., Singh, R.P., Suman, R.: Telemedicine for healthcare: capabilities, features, barriers, and applications. Sens. Int. **2**, 100117 (2021). https://doi.org/10.1016/J.SINTL.2021.100117

11. Manchanda, S.: Telemedicine-getting care to patients closer to home. Am. J. Respir. Crit. Care Med. **201**, P26–P27 (2020). https://doi.org/10.1164/RCCM.2020C5

12. Marins, F., Cardoso, L., Esteves, M., Machado, J., Abelha, A.: An agent-based RFID monitoring system for healthcare. In: Rocha, Á., Correia, A.M., Adeli, H., Reis, L.P., Costanzo, S. (eds.) WorldCIST 2017. AISC, vol. 571, pp. 407–416. Springer, Cham (2017). https://doi.org/10.1007/978-3-319-56541-5_42

13. Medina, M., et al.: Home monitoring for COVID-19. Clevel. Clin. J. Med. **87**, 1–4 (2020). https://doi.org/10.3949/CCJM.87A.CCC028. https://europepmc.org/article/med/32409432

14. Moreira, A., Guimarães, T., Duarte, R., Salazar, M.M., Santos, M.: Interoperability and security issues on multichannel interaction in healthcare services. Procedia Comput. Sci. (2022). https://doi.org/10.1016/j.procs.2022.03.096

15. Moreira, A., Guimarães, T., Santos, M.F.: A conceptual model for multichannel interaction in healthcare services. Procedia Comput. Sci. **177**, 534–539 (2020). https://doi.org/10.1016/J.PROCS.2020.10.074

16. Moreira, A., Miranda, R., Santos, M.F.: Health professional's decision-making based on multichannel interaction services. Procedia Comput. Sci. **184**, 899–904 (2020). https://doi.org/10.1016/j.procs.2021.03.112

17. Moreira, A., Santos, M.F.: Multichannel interaction for healthcare intelligent decision support. Procedia Compute. Sci. **170**, 1053–1058 (2020). https://doi.org/10.1016/j.procs.2020.03.074

18. Neslin, S.A.: Key issues in multichannel customer management: current knowledge and future directions. J. Interact. Mark. **23**(1), 70–81 (2009). https://doi.org/10.1016/J.INTMAR.2008.10.005. https://www.sciencedirect.com/science/article/pii/S1094996808000078

19. Neto, C., Ferreira, D., Abelha, A., Machado, J.: Improving healthcare delivery with new interactive visualization methods. In: Rocha, Á., Adeli, H., Reis, L.P., Costanzo, S. (eds.) WorldCIST'19 2019. AISC, vol. 932, pp. 537–546. Springer, Cham (2019). https://doi.org/10.1007/978-3-030-16187-3_52

20. Oliveira, D., Ferreira, D., Abreu, N., Leuschner, P., Abelha, A., Machado, J.: Prediction of covid-19 diagnosis based on openehr artefacts. Sci. Rep. 2022 12:1 **12**, 1–13 (2022). https://doi.org/10.1038/s41598-022-15968-z. https://www.nature.com/articles/s41598-022-15968-z

21. Oliveira, D., et al.: Openehr modeling: improving clinical records during the covid-19 pandemic. Health Technol. **11**, 1109–1118 (2021). https://doi.org/10.1007/S12553-021-00556-4/FIGURES/9

22. Rogers, L.C., Lavery, L.A., Joseph, W.S., Armstrong, D.G.: All feet on deck-the role of podiatry during the covid-19 pandemic: preventing hospitalizations in an overburdened healthcare system, reducing amputation and death in people with diabetes. J. Am. Podiatr. Med. Assoc. (2020). https://doi.org/10.7547/20-051

23. Stojković, D., Lovreta, S., Bogetić, Z.: Multichannel strategy-the dominant approach in modern retailing. Econ. Ann. **61**(209), 105–127 (2016)

24. Ventola, C.L.: Mobile devices and apps for health care professionals: uses and benefits. P&T **39**(5), 356–64 (2014). http://www.ncbi.nlm.nih.gov/pubmed/24883008. http://www.pubmedcentral.nih.gov/articlerender.fcgi?artid=PMC4029126

25. Wang, X., Zhang, Z., Zhao, J., Shi, Y.: Impact of telemedicine on healthcare service system considering patients' choice. Discrete Dyn. Nat. Soc. **2019** (2019). https://doi.org/10.1155/2019/7642176

Machine Learning In Healthcare

Steps Towards Intelligent Diabetic Foot Ulcer Follow-Up Based on Deep Learning

António Chaves[✉][iD], Regina Sousa[iD], António Abelha[iD], and Hugo Peixoto[iD]

ALGORITMI/LASI, University of Minho, Braga, Portugal
{antonio.chaves,regina.sousa}@algoritmi.uminho.pt,
{abelha,hpeixoto}@di.uminho.pt

Abstract. Diabetes is a chronic disease that affects the effective production of insulin in an individual. This incapacity leads to great damage to the cardiovascular system as well as the nervous system. Unfortunately this is a very present disease in today's population. Indeed, global diabetes prevalence is estimated to be between 9,5% and 10,5%. Diabetic patients have a need for constant monitoring and evaluation by the healthcare professional whenever diabetic foot wounds show symptoms of infection and ulceration. The high number of patients with this diagnosis makes follow-up a problem for health professionals as well as for the patient. Lack of communication and access to health care are major contributing factors to lower extremity amputations, high mortality and morbidity interventions. In order to solve this gap, the present work presents an architecture for the development of a collaborative and decision support tool, between not only health professionals but also patients, capable of rapidly and automatically identifying, assessing and treating ulcer and symptoms of the pathology. This automation will be implemented through classification models with Deep Learning.

Keywords: Diabetes · Computer Aided Diagnosis · Deep Learning · Ulcer Classification · Application Development

1 Introduction and Contextualization

Diabetes, a chronic disease that appears when the pancreas does not efficiently produce insulin or when the body is unable to utilize the insulin produced. Insulin is a hormone that deals with the regulation of blood sugar, and when uncontrolled for any reason it gives rise to an event of hyperglycemia (increased blood sugar). This is one of the most common effects of uncontrolled diabetes and over time leads to major damage to the cardiovascular system as well as the nervous system [1,2].

The classification of this pathology is divided into two types: Type 1 Diabetes and Type 2 Diabetes. Type 1 diabetes is associated with a deficit in insulin production and is treated by the daily administration of insulin to the body. Symptoms that may appear include excessive urine excretion, thirst, constant

ICST Institute for Computer Sciences, Social Informatics and Telecommunications Engineering 2023
Published by Springer Nature Switzerland AG 2023. All Rights Reserved
J. M. Machado and H. Peixoto (Eds.): AISCOVID 2022, LNICST 485, pp. 81–90, 2023.
https://doi.org/10.1007/978-3-031-38204-8_7

hunger, weight loss, vision changes, and fatigue. These symptoms can occur suddenly or not at all [3]. Type 2 diabetes, on the other hand, is associated with the inefficient use of insulin produced by the body. A large proportion of diabetes diagnoses are related to type 2 [4]. These are more easily identifiable because the patients complain a lot of body weight gain. For both types early diagnosis can be made through affordable tests that calculate blood sugar levels [5]. The treatment of diabetes involves diet and physical activity along with lowering blood glucose and the levels of other known risk factors that damage blood vessels [6].

According to the world health organization the treatment of diabetes should include blood sugar control, for example with oral medication, blood pressure control, screening and treatment of retinopathy (which causes blindness), blood lipid control, and not least foot care. This last point is one of the most important since Diabetic Foot Ulcers (DFU) are one of the most common occurrences in diabetic patients due to lower limb nerve damage and reduced blood flow in the area. To this end, patients should maintain patient self-care by maintaining foot hygiene, seek professional care for ulcer management, and have their feet examined regularly by healthcare professionals [2]. In this way Lower Extremity Amputations (LEA), which itself is associated with high morbidity and mortality in patients, may be decreased. In order to minimize the risk of LEA, careful and thorough monitoring of the lower limbs is necessary [7].

The main objectives of this study are the understanding of Artificial Intelligence implementations capable of supporting decision making and analyzing images related to possible DFU complications. Primarily, the concerning topics surrounding the matter will be explained, as well as the supporting evidence for the importance of the present study, followed by a state of the art review on architecture and neural network models chosen across different implementations. Lastly, the present work will present a proposed architecture for developing a tool for implementing a Decision Support System (DSS) capable of reviewing images submitted by DFU users.

2   Background

To achieve greater knowledge over the topic covered hereby, it is of great importance to understand some major topics, that this manuscript covers. First, diabetes and wound classification importance and struggles, making decision support systems an important step to achieve more efficient patient treatments. One of the most up to date technologies applied in the healthcare domain is Machine and Deep Learning and more specifically CNN.

2.1   Diabetes and Wound Classification

Diabetes is a chronic illness which, over time, leads to major damage to the body's cardiovascular and nervous system and is estimated to have been the direct cause of death of 6.7 million people in 2021, making it one of the top

10 leading causes of death in adults worldwide. Global diabetes prevalence is estimated to be between 9,5% and 10,5% of the population which amounts to 500 million cases, a number which has been steadily growing for the past two decades [8, 9].

Severe cardiovascular and nervous damage on a patient's body can result in poor wound healing, especially when present in the body's extremities. The detection of DFUs is usually a time consuming process done by experts and its correct classification and early detection detrimental in the reduction of LEA, which increase morbidity and mortality among diabetic patients.

2.2   Clinical Decision Support Systems

Clinical decision support systems (CDSS) are computerized frameworks implemented in order to improve healthcare delivery by enhancing medical decisions. To achieve this goal, the CDSS uses clinical knowledge that is built into the system which is used to analyze and explore data in order to discover patterns that may be useful for decision making, through Machine and Deep Learning techniques [10].

2.3   Deep Learning

Deep Learning is a subset of Machine Learning - and consequently Artificial Intelligence - aimed at automatically learning from knowledge without being explicitly programmed [11]. It differentiates itself from traditional ML techniques by applying successive layers of representation, often called Neural Networks, term derived from human physiology due to the similarity to our understanding of the brain. [12] The interest in Deep Learning has been continuously growing due to its success in Natural Language Processing and Image Recognition tasks, among others [13].

Up until 2012, Machine Learning algorithms made up most of the modern era solutions in the implementation of image recognition in computer vision. This was due to the fact that training Deep Learning methods was deemed complex and time consuming task and needed very large input quantities and computing power [14] in its study and contribution to an image classification competition and the astonishing results obtained shifted the attention to the use of Convolutional Neural Networks for the task. The author proves at the time that CNN can set record breaking metrics in image recognition and some ground truth needs for the success of the implementation of such methodology. First and foremost, Deep Learning models must be trained with large scale datasets. The specificity of some image recognition tasks - as is the reviewed DFU classification problem - and the lack of quality datasets may impose early constraints to a model's classification success rate. In order to minimize this issue, and to prevent the occurring of over-fitting issues, two techniques are usually employed. The first, Data Augmentation, is a simple task of converting each image in a dataset by applying a range of operations, such as rotation, pixel shifting and crop, to artificially increase the sampling size. This process can be automatically generated and is usually computationally inexpensive. The second relies on the use of pre-trained models, which should already be able to classify some image properties before being fine-tuned, so that further training may be focused solely the specific features on the classification task.

2.4 Convolutional Neural Networks

Convolutional Neural Networks are a subset Artificial Neural Networks, making use of the same neuronal architecture in order to self-optimize through learning. The main differences between CNN and ANN are the stacked layers that form the model, and their application to pattern recognition in images. The recognition of simpler defining aspects of images and their inclusion in the architecture allow for more precise image recognition tasks requiring fewer parameters for a correct model setup. CNNs are composed of three different types of layers: convolution, pooling and fully connected (FCL) layers. The first two serve the purpose of feature extraction, while FCL maps the outputs generated by the former into a result such as classification [15,16].

3 State of the Art

The prevalence of diabetes worldwide, along with technological progress and computer aided diagnosis have resulted in new viewpoints to help aid segmentation and classification in diabetic foot ulcers.

The use of Neural Networks comes as a successor to more traditional computer vision and machine learning methods. More specifically, Convolutional Neural Networks have been directly associated with image recognition tasks [17] and are the most common subject of research within the realm of automatic DFU diagnosis. Recent research in the subject can be highlighted in three categories: wound segmentation and classification algorithms and architectural design for implementation of related applications.

The authors in [18,19] respectively propose architectures based on the MobileNetV2 and MobileNet Convolutional Neural Networks for wound segmentation which substitute convolutional layers with depth-wise separable convolutional layers. It exponentially decreases computational cost compared to the traditional convolutional layers and suitable for applications where computing resources are limited with no observable trade-off in final results.

[20,21] utilize Encoder-Decoder based CNN models in their research, achieving state of the art scores in wound region mapping (Intersection over union and Data-based Dice). This NN architecture are mostly implemented due to their capability in data dimensionality reduction, noise suppression and data reconstruction. [22] Both studies make use of controlled images even though they differ in image quality sampling techniques. The first proposed the preprocessing of images by applying several augmentation techniques in the datasets supplied for model training while the second physically places a ruler with color markup in order to normalize color and enhance the precision of wound depth calculations.

While this may defeat the purpose of implementing a telemedicine application due to the controlled nature of image capture required, it shifts some attention to wound depth and size calculations, which may be difficult to infer, especially when keeping track of multiple stages of the same wound.

[23] proposes a binary classification method for DFU segmentation based on traditional CNN layers, with an AUC performance at 96%. The architecture of this method is split into three main sections, namely traditional GoogLeNet layers for cropping images of skin patching and normalization before transferring them to parallel convolutional layers for multi-level feature extraction followed by fully connected layers and a SoftMax-based output classifier.

Although not reporting the best metrics in reviewed literature, [24] offers good insight on a possible architecture for a fully working mobile platform consisting of a web application and a dedicated server for image processing and classification. Furthermore, the developed Multi-Label CNN Ensemble can classify most complications related to DFU such as infections and exudate.

4   Results

This study's goals can be divided into two main categories: an interoperable telemedicine application aimed at enhancing patient-doctor approximation, for rapid diagnosis of severe diabetic complications and a DFU segmentation framework based on Deep Learning, for rapid wound classification and medical decision support. As per noticed in reviewed literature, the implementation of a production ready system for DFU classification still faces the major problem of dataset suitability.

Model training requires a vast amount of records to be able to correctly serve its purpose. Most datasets observed in reviewed studies were imbalanced and lacked dimension and even when applying artificial augmentation were still far from desired proportions. These must also be backed by a manual classification done by professionals, a time-consuming task which requires cooperation from specialized DFU physicians. The heterogeneity of image capture devices will also impose a challenge to the model's classification prediction. Different devices, illumination settings and camera angles are all external factors to take into consideration.

Lastly, the implementation of the system is dependent on the patients' ownership of a smartphone or tablet device and its availability to run on different types of operating systems.

4.1   Proposed Architecture

The architecture proposition was based on [24] and [25] and is comprised of the following components:

- **Data Sources:** Different sources for data gathering for model training and testing;

- **Deep Learning Algorithm:** A Deep Learning Model capable of classifying submitted images of DFU, obtained from the optimization of a selected pre-trained algorithm;
- **Database:** Database for information storage. With patient permission, stored images may be supplied into the Deep Learning Model for further training and improvement on recognition tasks;
- **Back-end Server:** The architecture's business layer, a server for application login management and request routing;
- **Mobile Application:** Intended for patient's use, this part of the presentation layer should allow for image capture and submission as well as over time tracking of personal information and medical advice;
- **Web Application:** Management tool for physicians which allows them to review patient submitted images, along with the automatically generated classification and access to patient history.

The following Fig. 1 presents the applications components and their interactions.

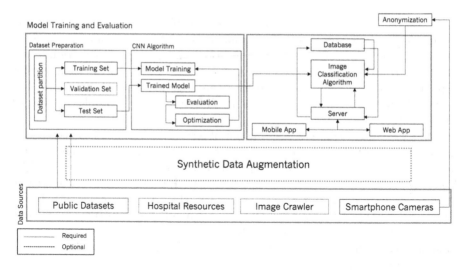

Fig. 1. Proposed architecture.

In order for a complete sample gathering of data, the combination of multiple data sources is optimal, so long as the dataset's content is balanced. The combined data gathered through public datasets and partner hospitals' own image databases can be run through an automatic Synthetic Data creation process so that the initial training and test data sample can be artificially increased. Healthcare facilities' data sources, which collect data for every patient making it a powerful tool in decision making, [26] can be an empowering factor in the image classification accuracy, in part due to their complete manual labelling and the opportunity to corroborate DFU with other types diagnosis. For example, DFU infections are usually difficult to diagnose without the support of specific blood tests.

This sample is then split in three subsets, for model training, validation and testing. The model's training process is recurrent until the error margin in testing images is deemed sufficient. The computational power required for a full training of DL architectures as well as the impact of the images' diverse characteristics can be diminished through the adoption of a pre-trained network, such as ImageNet, which allow an increase of the more specific local learning rate [27].

As is suggested, the architecture's back-end server is the core structure of the application and has a significant importance in request handling, database access, authentication and security. The application's end goal architecture relies on the centralized deployment of the back-end server and classification algorithm and, as such, the idea of a micro service implementation arises. This decision needs to be assessed before implementation and its analysis is substantially reliant on the amount of potential healthcare partners and patients. While scalability must be addressed, a monolithic architecture may be in order if survey data shows the number of potential users not to be a deciding factor also maintaining a lower relative computational cost and averaging faster response times [28].

The heterogeneity of nowadays users' devices implicitly guides the development of the mobile application into cross-platform ready development frameworks. The excessive cost of native development does not compensate for the drawbacks of cross platform such as limited access to functionality - as long as smartphone camera access is granted - and poorer performance.

User submitted images, gathered directly from personal devices, are sent for classification purposes through the designated Back-end Server routes. Their response should be quickly presented to the user and stored for user history and comparison. An important aspect of user images is their usefulness for further model training although subject to user permission for personal image use.

5   Discussion

The suggested architecture is based on [24]'s contribution, however, the suggestion of a embedded DL model within the Mobile Application, seems to be far from desired, especially taking into consideration modern era smartphone processing power. The trade off between performance metrics when comparing computer and smartphone systems is still noticeable [29] and should only be considered as a last resort for implementation. The pinpointed advantages of the embedded model such as offline usability and better responsiveness when compared to the use of an internet connection are still far outweighed by a 10% drop off in performance metrics.

The improvement of the models classification should be done through data augmentation and transfer learning techniques and further fine tuning by adding user submitted images to the training dataset, not only increasing its size but also in the anticipation of shaping the models capability of DFU identification, diminishing the aforementioned external factors' influence. If training data is still deemed insufficient or having an unbalanced distribution, the combination of different datasets can be set in place. The concept of dataset merging for training in segmentation networks proves NN performance can be boosted and thus provide better results [30,31].

On another note, the application's success is also highly dependent on its adoption from healthcare services and patients alike as recent cybersecurity issues can have a detrimental impact in social and consumer trust.

6   Conclusions

Diabetes is undoubtedly one of the most common diseases in developed countries, and lower limb nerve damage, due to low blood flow in such areas, can lead to severe complications such as DFU. Being a chronic disease, contributions to long term treatment, prevention, patient follow-up as well as better and more reliable treatment decisions are of great importance. In this study a framework for the implementation of a fully interoperable application capable of automatic DFU classification for rapid assessment is proposed. Indeed, this architecture has the potential to shift the paradigm of the treatment of severe diabetic complications, with an end goal of improving patients' lives. Main contributions vary from recognizing the main obstacles towards implementation to provide adequate solutions for these issues. Furthermore, the proposed architecture paves the way for the fulfillment of the DL model's training and optimization. Its design is scalable and modular, proposing a cross-platform framework with web and mobile capabilities settled in incremental development and overall usability.

Acknowledgements. This work has been supported by FCT—Fundação para a Ciência e Tecnologia within the R&D Units Project Scope: UIDB/00319/2020. The grants of Regina Sousa and António Chaves are supported by the project "Integrated and Innovative Solutions for the well-being of people in complex urban centers" within the Project Scope NORTE-01-0145-FEDER-000086.

References

1. Narres, M., et al.: Incidence of lower extremity amputations in the diabetic compared with the non-diabetic population: a systematic review. PLoS ONE **12**(8), e0182081 (2017). https://doi.org/10.1371/journal.pone.0182081
2. Collaboration, E.R.F.: Diabetes mellitus, fasting blood glucose concentration, and risk of vascular disease: a collaborative meta-analysis of 102 prospective studies. Lancet **375**(9733), 2215–2222 (2010)
3. Atkinson, M.A., Eisenbarth, G.S., Michels, A.W.: Type 1 diabetes. Lancet **383**(9911), 69–82 (2014)
4. Coffman, M.J., Norton, C.K., Beene, L.: Diabetes symptoms, health literacy, and health care use in adult Latinos with diabetes risk factors. J. Cult. Divers. **19**(1) (2012)

5. Chatterjee, S., Khunti, K., Davies, M.J.: Type 2 diabetes. Lancet **389**(10085), 2239–2251 (2017)
6. https://www.who.int . Accessed 15 Mar 2022
7. Morais, A., Peixoto, H., Coimbra, C., Abelha, A., Machado, J.: Predicting the need of neonatal resuscitation using data mining. Procedia Comput. Sci. **113**, 571–576 (2017). https://doi.org/10.1016/j.procs.2017.08.287
8. International Diabetes Federation: IDF Diabetes Atlas 10th Edition. International Diabetes Federation (2021)
9. Saeedi, P., et al.: Global and regional diabetes prevalence estimates for 2019 and projections for 2030 and 2045: results from the international diabetes federation diabetes atlas, 9th edition. Diabetes Res. Clin. Pract. **157**, 107843 (2019). https://doi.org/10.1016/j.diabres.2019.107843
10. Neto, C., Brito, M., Lopes, V., Peixoto, H., Abelha, A., Machado, J.: Application of data mining for the prediction of mortality and occurrence of complications for gastric cancer patients. Entropy **21**(12), 1163 (2019). https://doi.org/10.3390/e21121163
11. Dargan, S., Kumar, M., Ayyagari, M.R., Kumar, G.: A survey of deep learning and its applications: a new paradigm to machine learning. Arch. Comput. Methods Eng. **27**(4), 1071–1092 (2019). https://doi.org/10.1007/s11831-019-09344-w
12. Reinolds, F., Neto, C., Machado, J.: Deep learning for activity recognition using audio and video. Electronics **11**(5), 782 (2022). https://doi.org/10.3390/electronics11050782
13. Chollet, F.: Deep Learning with Python. Manning Publications, New York (2018)
14. Krizhevsky, A., Sutskever, I., Hinton, G.E.: ImageNet classification with deep convolutional neural networks. Commun. ACM **60**(6), 84–90 (2017). https://doi.org/10.1145/3065386
15. O'Shea, K., Nash, R.: An Introduction to Convolutional Neural Networks (2015)
16. Yamashita, R., Nishio, M., Do, R.K.G., Togashi, K.: Convolutional neural networks: an overview and application in radiology. Insights Imaging **9**(4), 611–629 (2018). https://doi.org/10.1007/s13244-018-0639-9
17. Szegedy, C., Ioffe, S., Vanhoucke, V., Alemi, A.: Inception-v4, inception-ResNet and the impact of residual connections on learning. In: AAAI Conference on Artificial Intelligence (2016)
18. Wang, C., et al.: Fully automatic wound segmentation with deep convolutional neural networks. Sci. Rep. **10**(1) (2020). https://doi.org/10.1038/s41598-020-78799-w
19. Liu, X. et al.: A framework of wound segmentation based on deep convolutional networks. In: 2017 10th International Congress on Image and Signal Processing, BioMedical Engineering and Informatics (CISP-BMEI) (2017). https://doi.org/10.1109/cisp-bmei.2017.8302184
20. Mahbod, A., Ecker, R., Ellinger, I.: Automatic Foot Ulcer segmentation Using an Ensemble of Convolutional Neural Networks (2021)
21. Chino, D.Y.T., Scabora, L.C., Cazzolato, M.T., Jorge, A.E.S., Traina-Jr., C., Traina, A.J.M.: Segmenting skin ulcers and measuring the wound area using deep convolutional networks. Comput. Methods Programs Biomed. **191**, 105376 (2020). https://doi.org/10.1016/j.cmpb.2020.105376
22. Ferreira, D., Silva, S., Abelha, A., Machado, J.: Recommendation system using autoencoders. Appl. Sci. **10**(16), 5510 (2020). https://doi.org/10.3390/app10165510

23. Goyal, M., Reeves, N.D., Davison, A.K., Rajbhandari, S., Spragg, J., Yap, M.H.: DFUNet: convolutional neural networks for diabetic foot ulcer classification. IEEE Trans. Emerg. Top. Comput. Intell. **4**(5), 728–739 (2020). https://doi.org/10.1109/tetci.2018.2866254

24. Shenoy, V.N., Foster, E., Aalami, L., Majeed, B., Aalami, O.: Deepwound: automated postoperative wound assessment and surgical site surveillance through convolutional neural networks. In: 2018 IEEE International Conference on Bioinformatics and Biomedicine (BIBM) (2018). https://doi.org/10.1109/bibm.2018.8621130

25. Brown, R., Ploderer, B., Da Seng, L.S., Lazzarini, P., van Netten, J.: MyFootCare. In: Proceedings of the 29th Australian Conference on Computer-Human Interaction (2017). https://doi.org/10.1145/3152771.3156158

26. Martins, B., Ferreira, D., Neto, C., Abelha, A., Machado, J.: Data mining for cardiovascular disease prediction. J. Med. Syst. **45**(1), 1–8 (2021). https://doi.org/10.1007/s10916-020-01682-8

27. Anwar, S.M., Majid, M., Qayyum, A., Awais, M., Alnowami, M., Khan, M.K.: Medical image analysis using convolutional neural networks: a review. J. Med. Syst. **42**(11), 1–13 (2018). https://doi.org/10.1007/s10916-018-1088-1

28. Al-Debagy, O., Martinek, P.: A comparative review of microservices and monolithic architectures. In: IEEE 18th International Symposium on Computational Intelligence and Informatics (CINTI), pp. 000149–000154 (2018). https://doi.org/10.1109/CINTI.2018.8928192

29. Suriyal, S., Druzgalski, C., Gautam, K.: Mobile assisted diabetic retinopathy detection using deep neural network. In: 2018 Global Medical Engineering Physics Exchanges/Pan American Health Care Exchanges (GMEPE/PAHCE) (2018). https://doi.org/10.1109/gmepe-pahce.2018.8400760

30. Kemnitz, J., Baumgartner, C.F., Wirth, W., Eckstein, F., Eder, S.K., Konukoglu, E.: Combining heterogeneously labeled datasets for training segmentation networks. In: Shi, Y., Suk, H.-I., Liu, M. (eds.) MLMI 2018. LNCS, vol. 11046, pp. 276–284. Springer, Cham (2018). https://doi.org/10.1007/978-3-030-00919-9_32

31. Srinivas, K., Gale, A., Dolby, J.: Merging datasets through deep learning (2018)

Recommendation of Medical Exams to Support Clinical Diagnosis Based on Patient's Symptoms

Cristiana Neto[1] , Diana Ferreira[1] , Hugo Cunha[2], Maria Pires[2],
Susana Marques[2], Regina Sousa[1] , and José Machado[3]([⊠])

[1] Algoritmi Research Center, University of Minho, 4710 Braga, Portugal
{cristiana.neto,diana.ferreira,regina.sousa}@algoritmi.uminho.pt
[2] University of Minho, Campus Gualtar, Braga 4710, Portugal
{a84656,a86268,a84167}@alunos.uminho.pt
[3] Department of Informatics, University of Minho, 4710 Braga, Portugal
jmac@di.uminho.pt

Abstract. Nowadays, it is essential that the error in the decisions made by health professionals is as small as possible. This applies to any medical area, including the recommendation of medical exams based on certain symptoms for the diagnosis of diseases. This study aims to explore the use of different Machine Learning techniques to increase the confidence of the medical exams prescribed by healthcare professionals. A successful implementation of this proposal could reduce the probability of medical errors in what concerns the prescription of medical exams and, consequently, the diagnosis of medical conditions. Thus, in this paper, six Machine Learning models were applied and optimized, namely, RF, DT, k-NN, NB, SVM and RNN, in order to find the most suitable model for the problem at hand. The results obtained with this study were promising, achieving high accuracy values with RF, DT and k-NN.

Keywords: Recommender System · Medical Exams · CRISP-DM · Classification

1 Introduction

The field of medicine is possibly the one that presents the greatest challenges in the integration of machine learning techniques. Starting from the basis of learning, these challenges lie in the nonexistence of datasets and in the difficulty of creating them due to inherent privacy issues. Clinical data are of a highly complex nature and are regularly incomplete and coming from various sources so they do not follow the same standards and records for the same problem may be incompatible [6].

The decisions made by health care professionals in a clinical diagnosis have direct impact on patients' treatment outcome. Due to the accelerated medical and technological growth, new options appear regularly, resulting in difficulties in

ICST Institute for Computer Sciences, Social Informatics and Telecommunications Engineering 2023
Published by Springer Nature Switzerland AG 2023. All Rights Reserved
J. M. Machado and H. Peixoto (Eds.): AISCOVID 2022, LNICST 485, pp. 91–100, 2023.
https://doi.org/10.1007/978-3-031-38204-8_8

choosing the most appropriate exams for patients [16]. Thus, the need to create recommender systems in order to assist professionals in the decision-making process becomes evident. In a generic way, a recommender system can be defined as a system that guides users in a personalized way to interesting or useful objects in a large space of possible objects or produces such objects as outputs [5]. In a medical perspective these objects can be the medical examinations that the patients will have to undergo and the users the health care professionals who will have to prescribe them.

One of the most important workflows in a hospital environment, that can be enhanced by the referred technologies, is the CMD (Complementary Means of Diagnosis) workflow. This workflow ranges from the request of the CMDs, to their scheduling and results reporting. Because of its importance, optimizing and enhancing this workflow is a key point in ensuring not only the proper functioning of the hospital institution but also a better healthcare deliver.

In this context, the current research has emerged, consisting in the development and exploration of machine learning algorithms for decision support in recommender exams for patients according to their symptoms. It should be noted that the recommendation is based on their symptoms only and not on their diseases, making the problem at hand more difficult since the intended goal is creating algorithms that can make a sort of intermediate diagnosis, managing to map the symptoms to the necessary exams without the need to take the intermediate step which is to think about which diseases the patient may have.

In this way, this study contributes to the optimization of the CMD workflow, since its successful implementation will reduce the prescription of unnecessary exams, as well as the overload of medical equipment, and consequently will improve the financial burden of the health institution.

The remainder of this paper is organized as follows: the next section presents an analysis of research papers related to the topic addressed in this study; Sect. 3 presents the methodology process carried out; Sect. 4 presents and discusses the results obtained; finally, Sect. 5 outlines the main contributions of this study and some ideas for future work.

2   Related Work

There are several articles and sources available on recommender systems in health care and on the respective best methods for mapping symptoms to diseases. This article has a greater goal and intends to go further by mapping the symptoms directly to the intended medical exams, not requiring a diagnosis beforehand. There is a greater scarcity of research in this particular area, and it is intended that the research carried out and exposed in this article can be an asset for future research work and a good basis for further advances.

Focusing first on general recommender systems in the health field, it is common knowledge that there are treatments for diseases that can be time consuming and a great monetary burden. To avoid this, there is a need for systems that can detect disease symptoms as quickly as possible and even help professionals make better choices when treating patients. Thus, recommender systems have already been proposed to predict risk factors (such as possible complications or future illnesses) that a certain patient with a chronic disease may face in the future [10,13].

In these particular systems, it is applied Collaborative Filtering, which recommends items to a user based on the following idea: "If users shared the same interests in the past, then they would have similar tastes". This approach can be interpreted in the context of these systems as follows: "Patients who share similar diseases and health status might face the same risk factors" [16]. Similarly, IBM's artificial intelligence machine, Watson Health, is already able to recommend suitable treatments for patients based on the outcomes of other patients and evidence-based medicine. According to IBM, 81% of healthcare executives who are familiar with Watson Health believe that it has a positive impact on their business [15]. This demonstrates that using technology and analytics has become increasingly important in healthcare.

The research and development of predictions in the domain of medical examinations is still quite early and has not been extensively explored. We argue that this is due to the specifics of bench-marking criteria in medical scenarios and the enormous context complexity of the medical domain. Risk perceptions towards data security and privacy, as well as trust in safe technical systems play a central role particularly in the clinical context. These aspects predominate in the acceptance of such systems.

3   Methodology

The benchmarking process followed the CRISP-DM (Cross Industry Standard Process for Data Mining) methodology, one of the most popular methodologies used in Machine Learning and Data Mining projects worldwide.

Figure 1 illustrates the methodology's life cycle, dividing it into six different stages: Business Understanding, Data Understanding, Data Preparation, Modelling, Evaluation and Deployment [8].

In the following subsections, each phase of the CRISP-DM will be discussed in more detail.

3.1   Business Understanding

Considering the complexity of medical data, as it is often unstructured, incomplete, non-standardized and stems from various sources or because large parts of data are not generated in a computer (as typical recommendations are) but stem from paper-based health-records that are often digitized afterwards, it is a challenge to provide accurate medical recommendations.

At this stage of the project, it is important to have a clear understanding of the main goals in order to ensure that the process is carried out rigorously and that an efficient recommendation system is therefore achieved. Hence, a set of goals were established for this study: to achieve a competitive advantage in the

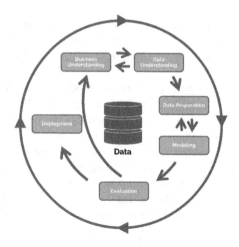

Fig. 1. Stages of the CRISP-DM Methodology.

evaluation of medical exams by health professionals; to be able to make personalized recommendations taking into account the type and number of symptoms; and to find the recommendation algorithm and parameterization that leads to the highest overall performance in the recommendation system.

3.2   Data Understanding

The medical sources used in this study are found in literature as open access for research purposes. Therefore, the data used in this study comes from the Disease Symptom Prediction [14] dataset, which is publicly available. The first dataset contains 4920 entries regarding 41 diseases and the symptoms experienced by different subjects suffering from that disease. There are 131 different symptoms in the dataset and for every disease, there is exactly 120 entries with combinations of symptoms experienced. This dataset also included an association of every symptom to a severity weight on a scale from one to seven. Due to the sensitivity of medical data and lack of datasets the mapping of the exams required to detect diseases had to be done manually through intensive research of reliable medical sources. Thus, a second dataset mapping every disease, present in the first dataset, was created. The number of medical exams per diseases ranges from two to seven, as it can be seen in Fig. 2. Some diseases are linked to very specific sets of medical exams while others require nothing more than a simple physical examination or a blood test to be detected by the professional. In the end, 102 different medical exams were compiled. Figure 3 displays the most common exams prescribed, where it is visible that prescribing blood tests and being physically examined by an health care professional is an important standard practice to understand and guide further diagnosis.

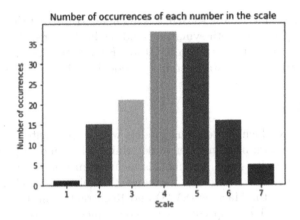

Fig. 2. Distribution of the severity of the diseases.

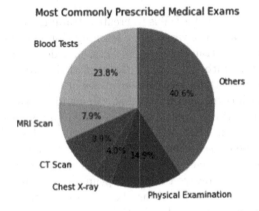

Fig. 3. Most Prescribed Medical Exams.

3.3 Data Preparation

Preparing the data is a crucial step to maximize the performance of the chosen models, therefore the chosen datasets had to be merged into one large dataset and the raw data properly treated to be able to be fed to the models afterwards.

The first step in this phase, consisted in the transformation of each symptom to a column using one-hot enconding. Consequently, it was associated the value 0 in the cases the symptom did not applied to the disease and the value 1 otherwise. After this step, since the public dataset used included a severity scale associated with the symptoms, each symptom in the dataset was mapped to its respective severity. Then, the constructed dataset that included the exams associated with each disease was also transformed using one-hot enconding and later merged with the previous dataset, using the disease as a common attribute in this operation.

After merging all the data, since it was intended to abstract the disease, which is the common factor of both symptoms and medical exams, this attribute was eliminated as it was not relevant to the study. Finally, the dataset was randomly divided using 80% of the data to train the models and 20% to test them.

3.4 Modeling

In this stage, six Machine Learning models were implemented and the hyper-parameters were optimized in order to determine which model performs best in the evaluation/results stage. The models included in this study were: Decision Tree (DT), Random Forest (RF), K-Nearest Neighbours (k-NN), Naïve Bayes (NB), Support Vector Machine (SVM) and Recurrent Neural Network (RNN). An exhaustive search over specified parameter values was performed for the first five algorithms.

Decision Tree. The goal of a DT is to create a training model that can predict the class or value of a target variable by learning simple decision rules inferred from the features of the training data. In DTs, in order to predict a class label for a record, we start with the rules at the root of the tree [8,12]. We compare the values of the root attribute with the values of the record's attribute, then we follow the branch corresponding to that value and afterwords we move on to the next node. For optimization purposes, we used Gini's index and entropy as criteria to measure which features should be in the nodes. The actual feature for each node can be chosen randomly from a distribution based on the metric of each feature or just by choosing the one with the best value, the thresholds picked in each node are always the most optimal. There is no pruning applied to the tree, however we tested limiting the tree growth to a max of 1, 10 or 20 nodes of depth as well as without a depth limit.

Random Forest. RF is a meta-estimator that uses the average of multiple DT classifiers, where each DT can be trained with a fraction of the dataset. Similarly to the DT classifier, the growth can be limited to 1, 10 or 20 nodes. The premise of this algorithm is that by using multiple tree classifiers with high randomness we can reduce the overall variance perceived in the resulting classification [11]. Since this is a meta-estimator, it is possible to define how many simple estimators to use. In this study, we evaluated the performance with 10, 20, 30, 50, 100, 200 and 1000 classifiers.

K-Nearest Neighbours. The k-NN classifier is a type of instance-based learning as it does not attempt to construct a general internal model, but simply stores instances of the training data. Classification is computed from a simple majority vote of the nearest neighbors of each point: a query point is assigned the data class which has the most representatives within the K nearest neighbors of the point.

In this study, the number of neighbors tested was 3, 5, 7, 11, 13, 15, 17, and 25. The value assigned to a query point when using uniform weights is computed from a simple majority vote of the nearest neighbors; however, when using weights based on distance, it assigns weights proportional to the inverse of the distance from the query point. The distance can be calculated using either the Euclidean distance formula or the Manhattan distance, and the search algorithm can use brute force or an acceleration structure such as a ball tree or KD-tree [2].

Naïve Bayes. The NB methods are a set of supervised learning algorithms based on Bayes' theorem with the "naive" assumption of conditional indepen-dence between every pair of features given the value of the class variable [1]. The main difference between each implementation of the NB classifier is how the likelihood of the features is computed.

Using the Gaussian formula, we can define the smoothing added to the variance as $1e{-}11$, $1e{-}10$ or $1e{-}9$ of the maximum variance reported. Using the Bernoulli formula, we can specify whether the algorithm should learn the prior probabilities before training. In addition, we can also specify the additive smoothing parameter as 0, 0.1, 0.2, 0.3, 0.4, 0.5, 0.6, 0.7, 0.9 or 1, which also works for the polynomial implementation of NB algorithm.

Support Vector Machines. SVMs are a set of supervised learning methods [4] whose goal is to find a hyperplane in an N-dimensional space, where N is the number of features, that clearly classifies the data points. Because SVMs are binary classifiers, N-binary classifier models had to be generated before they could be used in this context. One-vs-Rest is a heuristic method that fits each classifier against all the other classes [3] to achieve a multi-class classification.

Three different kernels were tested `poly`, `rbf`, `linear`, along with the opti-mization of the gamma value, which defines how far the influence of a single training example reaches the c value, which is the regularization parameter that controls miss-classification, and the class weight, which affects directly the c value.

Recurrent Neural Network. Neural Networks (NNs), commonly known as Artificial Neural Networks (ANNs) are a part of machine learning and are at the centre of deep learning algorithms. Their structure and nomenclature are based on the human brain, mirroring the communication between organic neu-rons. ANNs are comprised of node layers, containing an input layer, one or more hidden layers, and an output layer. With input data, weights, a bias (or thresh-old), and an output, each node represents a separate linear regression model. Before delivering information to the network's next layer, each node's output goes through a non-linear activation function. Otherwise, no data is transmit-ted to the network's next layer. Large volumes of training data are essential for neural networks to develop and enhance their accuracy over time [9].

Generally, neural networks perform tasks involving supervised learning, learning from data sets where the right answer has already been chosen. The networks then improve the accuracy of their forecasts by fine-tuning themselves to identify the proper response on their own. To achieve this, the network compares initial outputs with a given correct target. Depending on how much the initial outputs deviated from the goal values, a cost function is employed to adjust them. A crucial step in how a neural network learns a specific task is the back propagation across all neurons and connections to modify the biases and weights [7].

3.5   Evaluation

The goal of this study is to recommend a list of possible medical exams for a set of symptoms. The output of the neural network is not a list of medical exams. Because the network's output does not always converge to a binary list, the results must be processed before they can be evaluated. Starting with an array of booleans encoded with the one hot encoding standard, we apply a form of thresholding by averaging the maximum and minimum values in the resulting array.

In terms of evaluation, several metrics could be used, however when it comes to a medical recommender system, it is important to choose metrics that are truly useful and return relevant information. In this stage, we discussed the difference between the impact a false positive and a false negative, so we thought it would be interesting to create a new metric that shows simple statistics about the correctness of each answer.

Although the ultimate goal is to achieve 100% precision on every prediction, a 95% correct answer is considered extremely precise. With precision less than 95%, the error becomes overwhelming, so the average of the answers should not round this value. Hence, results less than 95% correctness should be accepted only in the context of watching the model evolve, as the distribution of the results is expected to shift from an average of 70% correct matches to greater than 95%.

It is important to keep in mind that the list of possible exams is not much more than 100 which means that a 90% correctness implies that the model recommended incorrectly over 10 exams, which might be catastrophic in a clinical setting depending on the patient's condition and on the healthcare professional's interpretation.

4   Results and Discussion

The results obtained in this study are compiled on Table 1, referring to the algorithm with the best parameters found by performing grid search. It can be observed that k-NN is the quickest model, taking only 3 s per fold and reaching 100% for both accuracy metrics. SVM is the second quickest with only 4 s per fold. RF and DT also achieved 100% for both accuracy metrics with an execution time of 6 and 10 s per fold, respectively. As for the NB algorithm, the highest accuracy was obtained applying the Bernoulli distribution. The real accuracy only achieved 82%, which means that in a universe of 1170 sets of tests, 86 were classified incorrectly. The incorrect classification of a set means that the recommendation system is not able to recommend the minimum required exams to detect the disease. On the other hand, the neural network's results are even lower and its training time is eighty times higher than k-NN's execution time.

Table 1. Best Results obtained using Grid Search and Cross Validation.

Model	Accuracy	Real Accuracy	Execution Time (s)
RF	100%	100%	30
DT	100%	100%	50
k-NN	100%	100%	15
NB (Bernoulli)	93%	82%	26
SVM	100%	100%	20
RNN (Optimal)	73%	62%	1200

5   Conclusion

Although recommender systems in medicine have made significant progress in recent years, continuous innovation and improvement are still required. Currently, there is a high demand for technological assistance for healthcare professionals in order for them to make the most accurate and error-free decisions possible. This study focused mostly on the implementation of different algorithms into the proposed recommender system, to serve as a launching point for future research in the field of health care, particularly, in medical exams. We discovered that using models such as RF, DT, and k-NN has great potential in this case, with an accuracy close to 100%. We argue that because of the shape and distribution of the data, these results must be carefully understood, and the way in which accuracy metrics are implemented in this situation should also be considered.

This study demonstrates that it is possible to combine human expertise (medical knowledge hidden in past decisions on the datasets under use) with computational power (artificial intelligence algorithms) to improve health care and provide a comprehensive recommendation with all of the necessary medical exams to detect a set of diseases that might be manifesting in the patient. In this case, it is advantageous to recommend as many medical exams as necessary to determine what is causing the symptoms; thus, the results are very satisfactory because the bare minimum of necessary tests is always recommended. Furthermore, the accuracy metrics developed in this study ensure that it addresses the previously mentioned concern and explains the high results obtained. Ideally, the models chosen to perform the benchmark on this study should be applied to a more diverse and realistic database, in this scenario it is expected that the RNN would perform better given the increase in the amount of data.

In the future, it would be interesting to apply the models to larger datasets to verify the generalization of the models and to improve professional criticism and patient health.

Acknowledgements. This work has been supported by FCT—Fundação para a Ciência e Tecnologia within the R&D Units Project Scope: UIDB/00319/2020. Diana Ferreira and Cristiana Neto thank the Fundação para a Ciência e Tecnologia (FCT) Portugal for the grants 2021.06308.BD and 2021.06507.BD, respectively. The grant of Regina Sousa is supported by the project "Integrated and Innovative Solutions for the well-being of people in complex urban centers" within the Project Scope NORTE-01-0145-FEDER-000086.

References

1. Naive Bayes. https://scikit-learn.org/stable/modules/naive_bayes.html
2. Nearest neighbors. https://scikit-learn.org/stable/modules/neighbors.html#neighbors
3. Onevsrestclassifier. https://scikit-learn.org/stable/modules/generated/sklearn.multiclass.OneVsRestClassifier.html
4. SVM. https://scikit-learn.org/stable/modules/generated/sklearn.svm.SVC.html
5. Adomavicius, G., Tuzhilin, A.: Toward the next generation of recommender systems: a survey of the state-of-the-art and possible extensions. IEEE Trans. Knowl. Data Eng. **17**(6), 734–749 (2005)
6. Calero Valdez, A., Ziefle, M., Verbert, K., Felfernig, A., Holzinger, A.: Recommender systems for health informatics: state-of-the-art and future perspectives. In: Holzinger, A. (ed.) Machine Learning for Health Informatics. LNCS (LNAI), vol. 9605, pp. 391–414. Springer, Cham (2016). https://doi.org/10.1007/978-3-319-50478-0_20
7. Chow, T.W.S., Cho, D.S.Y.: Neural Networks and Computing: Learning Algorithms and Applications, vol. 7. World Scientific (2007)
8. Ferreira, D., Neto, C., Lopes, J., Duarte, J., Abelha, A., Machado, J.: Predicting the survival of primary biliary cholangitis patients. Appl. Sci. **12**(16), 8043 (2022)
9. Maind, S.B., Wankar, P., et al.: Research paper on basic of artificial neural network. Int. J. Recent Innov. Trends Comput. Commun. **2**(1), 96–100 (2014)
10. Nasiri, M., Minaei, B., Kiani, A.: Dynamic recommendation: disease prediction and prevention using recommender system. Int. J. Basic Sci. Med. **1**(1), 13–17 (2016)
11. Neto, C., Brito, M., Lopes, V., Peixoto, H., Abelha, A., Machado, J.: Application of data mining for the prediction of mortality and occurrence of complications for gastric cancer patients. Entropy **21**(12), 1163 (2019)
12. Neto, C., Peixoto, H., Abelha, V., Abelha, A., Machado, J.: Knowledge discovery from surgical waiting lists. Procedia Comput. Sci. **121**, 1104–1111 (2017)
13. Patil, P.: Disease symptom prediction (2020). https://www.kaggle.com/itachi9604/disease-symptom-description-dataset
14. Patil, P.: Disease symptom prediction (2020). https://www.kaggle.com/datasets/itachi9604/disease-symptom-description-dataset
15. Stark, B., Knahl, C., Aydin, M., Elish, K.: A literature review on medicine recommender systems. Int. J. Adv. Comput. Sci. Appl. **10**(8) (2019)
16. Tran, T.N.T., Felfernig, A., Trattner, C., Holzinger, A.: Recommender systems in the healthcare domain: state-of-the-art and research issues. J. Intell. Inf. Syst. **57**(1), 171–201 (2021)

Author Index

© ICST Institute for Computer Sciences, Social Informatics and Telecommunications Engineering 2023
Published by Springer Nature Switzerland AG 2023. All Rights Reserved
J. M. Machado and H. Peixoto (Eds.): AISCOVID 2022, LNICST 485, p. 101, 2023.
https://doi.org/10.1007/978-3-031-38204-8

Printed in the United States
by Baker & Taylor Publisher Services